Foundations of Forensic
Document Analysis

Essentials of Forensic Science

Titles in the series:

Foundations of Forensic Document Analysis

Theory and Practice

Michael Allen

WILEY Blackwell

This edition first published 2016 © 2016 by John Wiley & Sons, Ltd

Registered office: John Wiley & Sons, Ltd, The Atrium, Southern Gate, Chichester, West Sussex, PO19 8SQ, UK

Editorial offices: 9600 Garsington Road, Oxford, OX4 2DQ, UK
The Atrium, Southern Gate, Chichester, West Sussex, PO19 8SQ, UK
111 River Street, Hoboken, NJ 07030-5774, USA

For details of our global editorial offices, for customer services and for information about how to apply for permission to reuse the copyright material in this book please see our website at www.wiley.com/wiley-blackwell.

Library of Congress Cataloging-in-Publication Data

Allen, Michael (Michael John), 1959- , author.
  Foundations of forensic document analysis : theory and practice / Michael Allen.
      p. ; cm. – (Essentials of forensic science)
  Includes bibliographical references and index.
  ISBN 978-1-118-64689-2 (cloth)......ISBN 978-1-118-72993-9 (paper)
  I. Title. II. Series: Essentials of forensic science (Forensic Science Society)
  [DNLM: 1. Documentation. 2. Forensic Sciences – methods. 3. Records as Topic. W 750]
  RA1147.5
  614'.1 – dc23
                                                                    2015006398

A catalogue record for this book is available from the British Library.

Wiley also publishes its books in a variety of electronic formats. Some content that appears in print may not be available in electronic books.

Cover image: © Hans Laubel/iStockphoto

Set in 10.5/13pt, TimesTenLTStd by SPi Global, Chennai, India.
Printed and bound in Malaysia by Vivar Printing Sdn Bhd

1   2016

Contents

6   Materials Used to Create Documents   145

7   Analytical Techniques Used in Document Examination   163

8   Altered and Tampered Documents   179

9 Indented Impressions   199

10 Dating Documents   213

11 Duties of The Expert   227

About the Author

Mike graduated from Keble College, Oxford University in 1981 with a degree in Physiological Sciences and went on to obtain an MSc in Forensic Science from the University of Strathclyde. In 2011 he completed his PhD with the University of Staffordshire having researched handwriting development in children.

Mike's forensic career began in 1983 in the Questioned Documents section of the Forensic Science Service laboratory in Birmingham, UK. In 1992, together with six colleagues, he helped to set up Document Evidence Limited to supply forensic document examination in the private sector to many police forces, other public bodies as well as lawyers and private clients. In 2008 Mike decided to semi-retire leaving Document Evidence but continuing to do some casework until finally retiring from that in 2013 having examined thousands of cases and given evidence in court on hundreds of occasions. He has been teaching document examination in several universities for a number of years and continues to do so.

Mike was Lead Assessor in Questioned Documents in the Council for the Registration of Forensic Practitioners from its inception and continued to play a role until its eventual closure in 2009. He has also been manager for the diplomas in Questioned Documents and Identity Documents for the Chartered Society of Forensic Sciences (previously the Forensic Science Society).

Series Foreword

Essentials of Forensic Science

The world of forensic science is changing at a very fast pace in terms of the provision of forensic science services, the development of technologies and knowledge and the interpretation of analytical and other data as it is applied within forensic practice. Practising forensic scientists are constantly striving to deliver the very best for the judicial process and as such need a reliable and robust knowledge base within their diverse disciplines. It is hoped that this book series will provide a resource by which such knowledge can be under-pinned for both students and practitioners of forensic science alike.

It is the objective of this book series to provide a valuable resource for forensic science practitioners, educators and others in that regard.

Professor Niamh Nic Daéid, FRSE
University of Dundee
Series Editor

Preface

What is document examination?

Forensic document examination is a wide ranging speciality that encompasses the examination of all aspects of document production. (The one examination type *not* involved is the examination of fingerprints on documents.) There are many aspects to document production, including handwriting and signatures, the examination of machine printed documents, alterations to documents, recovering information about how and when a document was produced, together with many other less frequently encountered problems – such as determining the sequence in which intersecting ink lines were written. The knowledge and experience required by the document examiner for handwriting comparisons thus ranges from matters such as the kinds of features to be found in handwriting, the determination of line fluency or the effects of age on handwriting, to an understanding of the components of ink and how they may be compared optically and chemically, to the composition of paper (potentially to the extent of determining how to identify tree species that make up a sheet of paper), to a knowledge of how mechanical devices such as typewriters, computer printers and printing machines work.

In other words, for a practitioner to be able to examine a document as a whole, rather than just some particular aspects of it, a broad, scientific training is invaluable.

In some countries the different subsets of the document examiner's scope are indeed divided up, for example there might be a handwriting expert, a forensic chemist to examine inks, an electron microscopist to look at the components in paper and a botanist to look at the tree species present. Traditionally, in the UK, many forensic document examiners deal with most of these sub-specialities. This has the advantage that a document can be considered from a number of angles by the same individual scientist who may then be best placed to integrate the information from different examination types to reach a more meaningful overall conclusion. For example, if a questioned agreement consisting of several pages is examined and contains typed entries, a signature and some handwritten annotations, then the document examiner has several lines of enquiry to follow whereas often the focus by non-experts would only be on the authenticity of the signature. A practitioner who only examined handwriting would therefore not necessarily be in a position to consider other lines of enquiry, such as page substitution or addition of entries at a later time.

Purpose of this book

The teaching of forensic science in universities in the UK has undergone significant change over the last 20 years, going from a subject taught at postgraduate level in a couple of universities (particularly those at the University of Strathclyde and Kings College, London), to undergraduate courses in many universities. This explosion of undergraduate courses has coincided with a number of excellent textbooks being published that cover all aspects of forensic science.

The content of general forensic science courses is inevitably divided up into various disciplines covering the mainstream topics such as biological material and physical evidence. Disciplines such as document examination therefore tend to form a small part of a much wider syllabus, and it is inevitable that the vast majority of students will not be seeking to pursue document examination as a career.

The teaching of some areas of forensic science has been made more difficult because the experience of the practitioner is such a valuable and essential part of the learning experience that it is not easy to impart knowledge to students other than in a detached 'textbook' fashion. And many that teach forensic science recognise the value that teaching by practitioners brings to the students' appreciation not just of the academic content but also the practical and court-related experiences that go with it.

So why write a textbook for students on this small part of their syllabus? While the majority of students will not become document examiners, the general forensic science student textbooks can only give a fairly brief (typically one chapter) outline of the subject. This book aims to extend that coverage primarily for students who want more than they can get from a general forensic textbook but less than they would get from one of the excellent books aimed more towards professional (especially training) document examiners.

Students inevitably have a different perspective on forensic science than that of practitioners, particularly as students need to acquire academic knowledge perhaps more than practical experience, although of course the two are closely entwined. So as a textbook aimed at students, the content of this book is different in some respects from that to be found in the practitioner texts. In addition, there is a need to not presume that readers have all of the basic knowledge needed to follow the diverse topics covered in the text. This in part is a reflection of the different subject backgrounds from which students come (which is translated into diverse degree subjects amongst practising document examiners). For these reasons, there are information boxes scattered throughout the chapters that contain what is intended to be helpful additional information for those not so familiar with some aspects of the subject.

Document examination is a very visual subject and it is inevitable that many explanations are enhanced by the use of images. In addition, it is probably the case that a good image reinforces the retention of the information in the text. For these reasons, there are plenty of diagrams and photographs to help make the words more readily understood.

Like all areas of forensic science, document examination produces a steady stream of published papers in scientific journals and forms the subject of conferences throughout the world. These rich sources of material are an important part of the subject at both academic and practitioner levels. For students, they provide an opportunity to enhance their academic understanding of the subject by digging deeper and deeper into the science behind the topics within the specialty. There are, therefore, plenty of references in the text to further reading for those minded to follow up aspects that they find particularly interesting.

In recognition of the continuing research developments and to enhance the content of the book there will be online updates detailing interesting new research papers and further worked examples to refresh the material available. To that extent, the book will always be a 'work in progress' in keeping with the steady accumulation of knowledge and technological changes over time. There are a number of topics currently that are of particular interest, including the attempts to harness the power of computers to assist the handwriting expert in a variety of contexts including automatic signature recognition (and the potential role of signatures as a biometric to identify a person) and giving some objective measures of handwriting features, the many different technologies applied to ink comparisons and a variety of conceptual approaches to dating ink on documents.

Structure of this book

The sub-topics that make up forensic document examination are in many ways fairly conceptually separate and this makes dividing the book up into self-contained chapters easier. However, there are elements that cross examination types and these relate especially to the procedures used when carrying out practical casework.

While this book is not intended to focus too heavily on those aspects that are better covered in books aimed at practitioners, it is essential that students are given a taste of what happens in the real world of casework. In order to achieve this each chapter finishes with two sections that first describe the kinds of information that are expected to be recorded by a practitioner working a case (note taking) and second some thoughts about how cases should be reported. While it was tempting to put the note taking into a separate chapter, as the principles that are involved are similar whatever the examination type being carried out, each different topic does require the recording of different sorts of information and hence each chapter will contain suggestions of what needs to be noted and why for the relevant topic.

At the end of most chapters there are worked examples that show how some mocked up cases could be examined in terms of notes taken and how they might be reported. The worked examples are intended to help fill the gap between *reading* and *doing* that will be familiar to many students. It is worth saying here that there are no universally agreed methods by which note taking should be done or examinations carried out. Nonetheless, the methods described in this book work and have stood the test of time for many practitioners.

As mentioned above, there are some books already available that cover forensic document examination or particular aspects of it and some of these are listed below. This book, therefore, aims to fill the gap between a chapter in a general forensic textbook and the more specialist books listed in the Further Reading section.

The author will be adding new references that are relevant as they are published and some more worked examples from time to time. Please visit qdbook.blogspot.co.uk for more details.

Further reading

Brunelle, R.L., & Crawford, K.R. (2003) *Advances in the Forensic Analysis and Dating of Writing Ink*, Springfield: Thomas Publisher.

Caligiuri, M. P., & Mohammed, L. A. (2012) *The Neuroscience of Handwriting: Applications for Forensic Document Examination*, Boca Raton: CRC Press.

Ellen, D. (2006) *Scientific Examination of Documents Methods and Techniques*, third edition, Boca Raton: CRC Press.

Hilton, O. (1992) *Scientific Examination of Questioned Documents*, Boca Raton: CRC Press.

Huber, R. A., & Headrick, A. M. (1999) *Handwriting Identification: Facts and Fundamentals*, Boca Raton: CRC Press.

Kelly, J. S., & Lindblom, B.S. (2006) *Scientific Examination of Questioned Documents*, second edition, Boca Raton: CRC Press.

Kelly, J. S. (2002) *Forensic Examination of Rubber Stamps: A Practical Guide*, Springfield: Charles C Thomas Pub Ltd.

Koppenhaver, K. M. (2007) *Forensic Document Examination: Principles and Practice*, New Jersey: Humana Press.

Levinson, J. (2000) *Questioned Documents: A Lawyer's Handbook*, London: Academic Press.

Morris, R. (2000) *Forensic Handwriting Identification: Fundamental Concepts and Principles*, London: Academic Press.

Acknowledgements

I have always been concerned over whether there was a gap in the market of excellent books that cover forensic document examination. However, I was convinced that for students, in particular, there was a need for a book showing how the practical side of the speciality was grounded in a robust theoretical framework. The journey from theory to practice is, in my experience, not always an easy one for students to make as they don't have the daily immersion in a subject that a trainee forensic document examiner would have, for example.

I therefore have been very fortunate to have the views of a recent student and now fully qualified document examiner responding to my question: Would this book have been helpful to you as a student? I am extremely grateful to Hannah Pocock for her enthusiastic help in making sure that this book keeps its focus on its intended audience and will, I hope, be beneficial to their studies. In addition, I am very grateful to Dr Andy Platt at Staffordshire University for looking over and suggesting some amendments particularly to Chapter 7. But, of course, I take full responsibility for the content of the book, not as daunting as taking responsibility for giving evidence in court as an expert witness, but daunting nonetheless knowing that attaining perfection and pleasing all readers is impossible!

I am very grateful to those at Wiley Blackwell who have helped me along the way in the, to me, new venture of book writing, in particular Rachael Ballard, Fiona Seymour, Audrie Tan, Delia Sandford and Rachel Roberts.

It goes without saying, but I will say it anyway, that without the cooperation of my family and especially my wife Karen, finding the time to write the book would have been that much more difficult.

About the Companion Website

Foundations of Forensic Document Analysis: Theory and Practice is accompanied by a companion website:

www.wiley.com/go/allen/forensicanalysis

The website includes:

Powerpoints of all figures from the book for downloading

1
Introduction

Forensic document examination, like all forensic specialties, is first and foremost based on knowledge. However, there are many other important aspects to the job that should not be overlooked because knowledge on its own is not enough to ensure the competence of experts. In this chapter these other aspects are described to give the reader some idea about these issues, which are easily overlooked but which are vital if the quality of forensic procedures is to be fit to be put before the courts.

1.1 Historical background

Just when and where writing started is not certain, but it has been around for thousands of years and probably first appeared in the eastern Mediterranean, at least partly driven by the need to record trading transactions among seafaring nations such as the Phoenicians – who may have been the first to create an alphabet.

Whatever its historical origins, once people started to write it was inevitable that others would start to abuse the written form for fraudulent reasons. In the intervening years, the criminal motivations have probably changed very little but the means to achieve them have changed beyond all recognition.

Document examination, and in particular handwriting examination, has been a recognised specialty in the context of the judicial systems of many countries for well over 100 years. Part of the reason for its early inclusion centres on the importance of handwriting, and in particular signatures, as a mark of agreement and endorsement to authorise various business and other transactions. The need for a third (independent) party to give an opinion about the genuineness, or otherwise, of disputed signatures and handwriting can readily be appreciated.

Foundations of Forensic Document Analysis: Theory and Practice, First Edition. Michael Allen.
© 2016 John Wiley & Sons, Ltd. Published 2016 by John Wiley & Sons, Ltd.
Companion Website: www.wiley.com/go/allen/forensicanalysis

As technology developed in the late nineteenth and throughout the twentieth century new problems for document examiners arose in tandem with the expansion of business and commerce across the world, and as a result much of the work of the expert is concerned with commercial transactions. Nonetheless, the domestic environment continues to produce its share of cases, from anonymous letters to ransom demands to murder and terrorist activities.

Other strands of document production have their own separate histories, such as the production of paper, the use of printing, advances in ink formulation and writing implements and the development of the typewriter and its eventual replacement by the computer printer. The many faceted work that faces the document examiner tasked with determining a document's authenticity has made the specialty a mainstream forensic discipline present in forensic science laboratories across the world.

In the early days of the specialty, textbooks on document examination were few and far between and they generally focused on handwriting and signature examination, but in 1910 in the USA the first book to draw the disparate examination types together into one place was written by Albert S. Osborn and entitled *Questioned Documents*. Since then a number of textbooks have been written, each one able to give more up-to-date information as methods have improved and developed.

While document examination is widely regarded as a mainstream forensic specialty, and certainly there is no disputing the need for experts in this discipline if cases involving documentation are to be prosecuted, one question that needs answering is: Are the underpinning foundations of document examination robust? Or put another way, can the courts rely on the evidence that forensic document examination provides (and that individual practitioners present in a given case)?

1.2   Is document examination a science at all?

Forensic science, by its high profile nature and the considerable public interest in the subject – both in the real world and in fiction, is perhaps one of the most scrutinised of scientific endeavours. Given the consequences that arise from it (fines, imprisonment and more depending on the country) it is of course quite right that all areas of forensic science should be able to justify themselves so that the public can be as sure as is humanly possible that the evidence presented to the courts is the best available.

And there is the first (and most intractable) problem – forensic science is a *human* endeavour – it does not exist in a world where uncertainty and error are somehow suspended in striving for absolute perfection and reliability. The possibility of error should be the single biggest factor influencing practitioners as they endeavour to maintain as high a standard as possible in all that they do, as they determine the evidence in a case, and especially when assessing the weight of their evidence. Most of forensic science ultimately comes down to interpreting evidence, and that is a cerebral process conducted by the expert, whatever the specialty, based on whatever evidence has been discovered and evaluated. Thus, using technology to detect, analyse and measure amounts of material (be it drugs in the body or DNA on clothing) is often just the foundation upon which the expert's opinion is based. There are instances when the technology may effectively be providing the expert evidence – such as identifying what a suspicious white powder is (of course, using the technology correctly is itself an endeavour requiring expertise). But expert evidence is human *opinion* evidence, not machine-generated data. Indeed, one of the most important factors that defines expert witnesses is that they are allowed to, indeed are encouraged to, express an opinion about the significance of their findings. Opinion evidence is almost forbidden from other categories of witness in many legal jurisdictions.

In this context, the specialty of document examination will be seen in the following chapters to have to admit that it does not always have many databases upon which to call when assessing evidence. The greatest focus of criticism of the specialty has generally been on handwriting and signature examination (Risinger et al. 1989). As we will see in this book, much work has been done by various researchers to address some of the criticisms and in so doing provide reassurance that the knowledge and processes that underpin the specialty of document examination are of sufficient reliability to justify their use. The capability of individual practitioners is a separate matter that also needs consideration.

In many areas of science, the use of computing power has transformed the methods and procedures used and it is not surprising that this is also true in document examination, particularly so in handwriting and signature identification. Perhaps one of the principal motivations for such an approach is to remove (or reduce) the human element of the expert's opinion and replace it with a mathematical (non-human) result based upon a de-personalised evaluation of the evidence. In Chapter 2 some consideration is given to the use of computers in handwriting examinations. The fact is, however, that despite considerable amounts of research into computer-based methods of assessing handwriting, no method has emerged to replace the human expert. At best, some of the findings of these research endeavours provide assistance to, but in no way yet replace, the human expert.

The reason for this is that of all of the 'things' that forensic practitioners examine (from paint to glass to body fluids), handwriting is unusual in being the constantly varying physical product of the human mind and body, unlike any other physical material that forensic science tries to examine. (Some of the closest relations are forensic phonetics and forensic linguistics, which seek to examine the human voice and the way that we use language, respectively, and forensic gait analysis, which assesses how we move as we walk.) Handwriting examination does not have the luxury of having invariant materials to look at, be they glass fragments, flakes of paint, or stains from biological fluids, the analyses of which do not have to cope with intrinsic natural variability let alone variability that is under human control.

It can readily be seen why technological solutions that address questions such as 'what is this thing made of' are less difficult to answer than questions such as 'who did this handwriting', for example, given that every piece of handwriting is unique and people may deliberately try to disguise their writing or else someone may try and copy their handwriting. How does a computer [operator] factor in even those basic issues since there are no global rules that dictate how good or bad a particular person is at writing (or how variable it is), disguising or copying?

The study of handwriting can currently only be carried out by human practitioners, albeit potentially with some assistance from computers that can provide some supporting information in some instances. The processes involved in handwriting comparison are described in Chapter 2. In some ways the requirements are really quite simple to describe, as in essence they require a forensic document examiner to undertake a lot of study around the subject and gain experience in examining handwriting from many people in many case situations to build up a personal database of experience and information. This may seem to be a cause for concern since this leads to experts forming opinions based on reasons that are not freely available in the public domain but are rather based on thoughts that occur in their heads. This misses the point that experts must be able to show they have followed appropriate methods (such as those described in Chapter 2) and they must be able to demonstrate and justify their opinions to others (such as the court). Any specialty that allowed practitioners to say 'This is my expert opinion, take it or leave it' would rightly be discounted. Ironically, the more technologically advanced the methods used by a forensic practitioner, the more there is an element of trust between their evidence and those using it, simply because the complexity of the technology is beyond the understanding of the lay person. Indeed, the actual *working* of a piece of equipment may not be fully understood by the person operating it, but the *results* obtained from it (from which the evidence is then derived) are of course understood.

Science can be defined as an intellectual and practical activity requiring the comprehensive study of the structure and behaviour of the world by observation and experiment. Looking at the elements of this definition in relation to handwriting, the *activity* of handwriting examination encompasses both intellectual (interpreting what is observed) and practical (observing and recording findings) aspects. The examination process is *comprehensive* (it is based on a thorough and complete process not focusing on isolated aspects). The relevant structure is in the handwriting (and an understanding of its physiological origins) and the behaviour is covered by an understanding of the capabilities of people when writing. The experimental dimension is given in the body of published knowledge that can be drawn on by practitioners. And careful observation is the single most important element of the examination process whatever the forensic specialty.

The notion that science somehow exists outside of human endeavour, in particular in a machine-based, infallible and statistically perfect world, is not only wrong, it is potentially dangerous precisely because the human elements of understanding and interpretation can be all too readily subsumed to a machine that then conveniently becomes the source of error (thereby allowing a practitioner to be absolved from any implied criticism when an error occurs). This diminishes the role of the (human) expert to the point where personal responsibility for the evidence placed before, say, a court is deflected to machines.

Looking at this another way, there is an expectation that human forensic practitioners are infallible when presenting their evidence. This is as unreasonable as it is ridiculous. No aspect of human endeavour can live up to such a high level of pressure, not medical science, not computer science, not even the law.

The National Academy of Sciences report (National Research Council, 2009) into forensic science added another layer to this debate by insisting that *any* specialty should justify its methods *and* also require a process of ensuring that individual practitioners can demonstrate an appropriate level of competence. In other words, there is a (deceptively) simple two-stage process needed to make sure that the science is good and that the scientist is good, or more broadly, that the methods used in any forensic specialty are good and the practitioners are good (hence side-stepping the issue of just what constitutes science with all of the mental baggage that almost everyone attributes to it). Surprising to some might be the fact that even those specialties that are widely regarded as safest, from fingerprinting to DNA, are not immune from needing to demonstrate the theoretical and practical underpinnings of their practice.

Handwriting (with signatures) has come in for its share of attention in this wider debate and this has been very well summarised by Kirsten Jackson in Chapter 6 of the second edition of *The Scientific Examination of Questioned Documents* (Kelly & Lindblom, 2006). The standing of forensic evidence was tested in the US courts using what was often called the Frye test (named after a particular judgement in the USA) in which the concept of *general acceptance* of the methods and knowledge in a specialty amongst those working in the peer group was regarded as a reasonable approach to adopt. In other words, if most practitioners regarded a particular methodology acceptable then the courts would accept that as an adequate demonstration that it was sound.

In 1993, in the US Supreme Court, a decision was taken to consider this principle of general acceptance together with a different principle based on the idea that the court would accept evidence that was based on scientific or other specialised knowledge providing it was likely to assist rather than hinder the court and, crucially, it was left to the court to determine the acceptability (by questioning the experts) on a case-by-case basis. This was the so-called Daubert ruling.

These general principles then came to be applied to a case known in short-hand as Starzecpyzel in which the court described handwriting testimony as a technical skill rather than a science and called into question the underpinning of the subject. This has led to a number of studies (discussed in Chapter 2) to improve the published literature on the methods and reliability of handwriting and signature examinations in particular. Similar focus on improving the robustness of processes has occurred in other specialties. The net result has been a greater output of published materials aimed at demonstrating the underpinnings of all forensic specialties.

Specific cases and legal rulings do not apply to other countries and so these rulings did not have a direct influence in the UK. Nonetheless, forensic practice is a worldwide profession and it is wise that all practitioners should be mindful of developments elsewhere. There have been repercussions in the UK inasmuch as the legal authorities have looked at the standards behind expert evidence here too. In the UK a key role in this is played by the Forensic Science Regulator who is responsible for standards in forensic practice, working in conjunction with the practitioners in the various specialties.[1]

1.3   Quality assurance

The problematic nature of decision-making was highlighted in the previous section and its relevance to the forensic process is huge because forensic practitioners make many, many decisions during the course of their examinations. Depending on the specialty involved, the use of test results derived from various items of equipment will also need to be fed into the decision-making process. However, pieces of equipment, just like people, are also not infallible precisely because people build and maintain them.

Given these constraints, the notion of having another expert to check findings makes a lot of sense, since certain categories of error can readily be identified and corrected. Clerical errors are inevitably commonplace and having someone read over a report will reduce their occurrence – but not eliminate their possibility. To reduce the likelihood yet further, a second checker could be employed and even a third. This makes the point that all processes have to have a sensible limit, and having one or at most two checkers is a very fair and sensible way of reducing as close to zero as possible the probability of, say, clerical errors.

The request that an investigator makes of the forensic practitioner determines to a large extent what the expert will decide to do and, importantly,

---

[1] https://www.gov.uk/government/organisations/forensic-science-regulator.

not to do in the case. It is to be expected that a busy expert may misread or misunderstand what is required and this highlights a second purpose of any checking procedure, namely to make sure that the relevant questions have been addressed in the expert's report. This may seem uncontroversial, but it can cause problems if during a forensic examination evidence is uncovered that has not been asked for by the investigator but which may be relevant to the overall matter in hand. The expert can either ignore the non-requested evidence (but that might lead to a miscarriage of justice) or notify the investigator or, better still, put it into the report even if the investigator (or some other interested party) seeks to have it removed and, more likely still, refuses to pay for the extra time spent on the additional examination.

The primary reason for checking an expert's findings, however, is to get a second expert's view as to whether the conclusion (and the reasons leading to it) is reasonable and the weight of evidence expressed (opinion) is consistent with the outcome of the forensic examination given the circumstances of the case. The views of a second expert are clearly valuable since if two experts agree then it is more likely that the conclusion is robust.

However, there is one difficulty, and that relates to how experts in any specialty acquire their knowledge and experience. We all learn the vast majority of what we know and can do from others who have gone before. In a forensic practice context, that means gaining knowledge at, say, university and then being trained in a particular laboratory environment to gain experience of applying our knowledge. This can tend to produce a situation where a practitioner does what they have been taught and, in due course, passes that on to the next generation. If several organisations are able to carry out forensic examinations in a given specialty, it is likely that they all operate in slightly different ways, due to slight variance in practice advocated by the individual experts in each place, but also constrained by, for example, the availability of equipment. There is, therefore, the potential for institutional differences of approach in a given specialty, and indeed this does occur ('our lab does it differently to your lab'). In order to try to reduce the effect this might have on the consistency of evidence from different organisations, collaborative studies can be carried out that provide the same material for examination to those participating and the results obtained can then be compared and discussed. From such exercises, it is hoped that best practice (or good practice or, at least, highlighting bad practice) will emerge with a consensus view as to what methodologies are appropriate to given examination types.

Of course, practitioners can be tested to see how well they deal with such exercises. Testing is a normal part of most practitioners' work load. Tests can be declared (so that the practitioner knows it is a test) or undeclared (so-called blind trials). Declared trials tend to be much easier to arrange but they have the drawback that awareness of being tested does alter the 'psychology' of the situation with practitioners becoming more wary and looking for traps in the evidence, for example. Undeclared trials are better from this perspective since the practitioner treats them in a 'normal' manner, unaware that they are a test; but getting material into a laboratory with all of the administrative 'red tape' that is involved makes this a much less frequently used test procedure.

One particularly valuable form of testing is where experts in different laboratories are given the same test material and after completion the results are compared. This inter-laboratory regime is good at passing on good practice and should lead to common standards being applied so that the final users (investigators and the courts) obtain a reasonably uniform quality of result irrespective of which organisation they go to for their forensic services.

1.4   Standards in forensic document examination

There is much merit in the idea of determining and then publishing good practice guidelines in a forensic specialty for reasons of quality and consistency of evidence put before the courts. The highest level for such standards are the ISO standards published by the International Organisation for Standardisation (whose acronym varies in different languages so ISO was settled on as being similar to, but not identical with, any of the languages concerned). There is no ISO standard specifically for forensic practice, let alone document examination. The nearest standards that have been adopted are:

- ISO/IEC 17025 General requirements for the competence of testing and calibration laboratories, and

- ISO/IEC 17020 Conformity assessment – Requirements for the operation of various types of bodies performing inspection.

ISO 17025 is the standard that closest matches the function of forensic practice, especially laboratory-based examinations. ISO 17020 applies more to the crime scene and its inspection since there is less emphasis on analysis and interpretation at that point in an investigation. Having stressed the value of consistency and cooperation between organisations (not just those concerned with *forensic* practice) in the previous section, such cooperation has been formalised in the International Laboratory Accreditation Cooperation (ILAC), which publishes guidelines that help to achieve this, one of which, known as G19,[2] has the purpose of interpreting the ISO 17025 standard in a forensic laboratory context.

The process of conducting assessments of laboratories against these two ISO standards is managed in the UK by the United Kingdom Accreditation

---

[2] Guidelines for Forensic Science Laboratories available online at https://www.ilac.org/documents /g19_2002.pdf.

Service (UKAS). The assessment process is very detailed and looks at both the *management* of an organisation and at the *technical* aspects carried out by the practitioners within the organisation. The reasoning is essentially that *both* aspects must be fit for their intended purpose if an organisation is to function properly: in other words neither a well-run laboratory producing poor results, nor a technically competent but poorly organised laboratory, would comply with the standard. Much of the assessment process looks at records (paper-based or more often computer-based) of laboratory functioning covering typical business functions but with some emphasis on those that might impact on the technical side, for example the repair and maintenance records of equipment or the environmental control records in a DNA lab. The technical aspects involve the pieces of equipment used, the reliability of the results obtained from them and the interpretation made by the forensic practitioners. In parallel to this is an assessment of the staff capability and training needs and thus there is some focus on individual practitioners – not with a view to registering each individual as competent but to establish that the organisation properly supports staff and tests their competence appropriately (for example by using trial cases with known outcomes) so that only those practitioners that the *organisation* is satisfied are capable of dealing with particular cases will be allowed to do so.

Thus the ISO standards are generic and do not contain any information relating to specific specialties. ISO 17025 in particular is primarily focused on test results from a laboratory (with the emphasis very much on equipment-derived results) and has very little to say about the interpretation of findings that lead to expert opinion evidence. To fill the gap in specialty-specific standards, there are published guidelines in many areas of forensic practice that describe in general terms how to approach various types of examination. For example, there is SWG (Scientific Working Groups) DRUG for drug analysis and SWGDOC for document examination. The recommendations made by these Scientific Working Groups are available online[3] and provide step-by-step summaries of good practice derived from the combined experience of a number of practitioners.

Another similar set of standards covering many aspects of scientific work, including a number relating specifically to document examination, is published by ASTM International (previously known as the American Society for Testing and Materials), which again can be obtained online.[4]

Compliance with the recommendations in these various standards is a good starting point for practitioners, who can be reassured that the practical methods that they employ are in keeping with what others in the field regard as appropriate.

---

[3] SWGDOC at http://www.swgdoc.org/index.php/standards/published-standards.
[4] at http://www.astm.org/Standards/forensic-science-standards.html.

Crucially, however, compliance with a standard or recommended approach is not a guarantee that the results obtained in a particular case will be correct or interpreted correctly. Obviously, the implementation of the methods and the interpretation of the findings require human skills, and this is where the competence of *individual* practitioners becomes the central issue.

1.5   Competence of forensic practitioners

The courts in most countries are the final arbiters of who can and cannot give expert testimony. In most countries, the courts have received advice as to how they should go about this because forensic evidence is widely recognised as being particularly valuable in many cases in assisting the court in its deliberations. Three of the key concerns are: (i) the robustness of the knowledge underpinning the specialty, (ii) the competence of the individual practitioner in front of the court and (iii) the relevance of the evidence to the case. Point (iii) is very much outside the practitioner's remit, but demonstrating individual competence is something that is central to establishing a witness's credibility.

In many professions, ranging from doctors to lawyers to architects, there are schemes that are designed to allow individuals to obtain recognition of their ability to do their respective jobs. Typically, such schemes may involve some sort of testing. Attitudes to such testing and the need for it have changed significantly in recent years, not least in the aftermath of the trial of Dr Harold Shipman for the murder of some of his patients, which had the consequence that professionals could no longer guarantee the trust of the public simply by virtue of their professional standing in the community. In addition, a number of high profile court cases in which forensic evidence played a significant part highlighted the need for forensic practitioners to justify their important place in the legal system.

The UK government devised a register of experts who had demonstrated their competence and set up an organisation, the Council for the Registration of Forensic Practitioners (CRFP), to manage the scheme. From 1999 to 2009 the register grew to around 3000 experts from a wide spectrum of different specialties. Due to a number of pressures on CRFP, it then became unable to operate and disbanded. However, the process that was used to demonstrate competence is of interest here. Competence was focused explicitly on current casework as opposed to, for example, formal qualifications. The central element of the test of competence was a peer review by an experienced expert from the same specialty of some recent casework (rendered anonymous). The assessment looked at how the candidate approached the case, the methodology used, the interpretation of the results and data in the context of alternative hypotheses, and the writing of an appropriate report, all of which constitute the main requirements of a forensic examination in any specialty.

Following the closure of CRFP, the Chartered Society of Forensic Science (CSoFS) initiated a register of experts aimed primarily at practitioners who were not employed by the larger forensic organisations and who were concentrating on gaining accreditation against the relevant ISO standards, a process that requires a lot of time and effort and the cost of which for some practitioners (in the widest sense of the word) makes it difficult to justify. The registration process adopted by the CSoFS involves peer review of some casework but in addition requires a candidate to undergo a test of their technical knowledge in their specialty, a test of their knowledge of their wider forensic awareness in relation to more general matters such as the working of the courts, the interpretation of evidence and their professional responsibilities and duties, and finally a test of their technical competence in a mock case exercise. This rigorous process, if completed successfully by a candidate, will entitle them to be registered on the CSoFS register of experts.

There is, therefore, a lot of attention being paid to the quality of forensic evidence that is put before the courts, attention that is a reflection of the increasingly important role that forensic evidence plays in judicial systems around the world.

Organisations and individuals that achieve accreditation and registration may feel that they have done all that is humanly possible to demonstrate to others their competence. But there is one more matter that they need to be aware of and that is perhaps the most intractable – cognitive bias – the unintentional misuse and misinterpretation of information by all of us.

1.6 Cognitive bias

Another issue that needs to be addressed, aside from the need to demonstrate the validity of the methodology and the experience and ability of the individual practitioner in a given specialty, is the universal problem of just how human beings make decisions, an issue that is central to all our endeavours and which nowhere comes under closer scrutiny than in the courts. The notion that any human being is a completely objective, robotic calculator of information is, of course, absurd. It follows that everyone is influenced (consciously or unconsciously) by all manner of facts and information and bias and prejudice and these require extra effort and procedures in an attempt to overcome them (Kahneman, 2011). The legal profession is itself not immune from the same issues, and it is therefore not surprising that given the many pieces there are to most legal jigsaws, and the fact that the ultimate decision-makers (such as judges and juries) themselves cannot escape from these cognitive effects, there has to be an acceptance that misjudgements (in the widest sense) will occur. Whilst this may be difficult to accept, it is much more dangerous if participants in legal matters think and believe that they are above such human failings because, in reality, no one can be.

Once this is realised, then it is possible to start to put in place measures that can minimise these effects. One obvious starting point is to make sure that an expert's findings and conclusions are checked over by another expert (see Section 1.3 above). Cognitive bias and, more broadly, the ways in which people make decisions, has become a major area of study but has only more recently been picked up by the forensic community. Research is being published into the effects it might have and how to minimise them in a practical environment. For example, suitable management of the flow of information in casework can reduce an expert's exposure to irrelevant potential sources of bias (Found & Ganas, 2013). Of course, one component of a submission can never be overcome, namely the fact that the material is being submitted for forensic examination at all means that someone somewhere thinks that it is worthwhile and more often than not it is submitted to confirm a pre-existing suspicion. That is not to say that sometimes material will be sent in for forensic examination with a view to ruling out either a particular suspect or to discounting a particular version of events. In situations where forensic examinations are directly paid for, there is a further danger that an expert might be influenced by this financial aspect of the transaction.

The decision-making process is obviously related to the way in which an expert makes the examination in the first place, and in some areas of forensic practice that require an assessment and interpretation of patterns (such as handwriting, blood pattern analysis and fingerprints) the way that the expert literally visualises the evidence is crucial since focusing the eyes on one part at the expense of another may form another unintentional 'bias' of perception (Dyer et al., 2006).

It is clear then that the underpinning science and technology, the competence of individual practitioners and the ways that they carry out their tasks, are all active issues in forensic practice, and this is a very healthy state of affairs since complacency is unacceptable in such an important profession. These issues are easily overlooked by those studying and thinking of starting careers in these disciplines.

1.7   Training to be a forensic document examiner

Forensic document examination requires a number of skills that need to be combined to give a well-rounded education that will lead to a career in the specialty. The remaining chapters of this book are concerned with the knowledge needed. However, no amount of knowledge can make up for the benefits gained from experience, and because much of what the document examiner does requires high levels of interpretation, gaining experience is an element of the job for which there is no substitute. For a potential recruit into the discipline this poses a problem, namely how to get into a career for which experience counts so much when having little or no experience to start the ball rolling. In reality, most trainee examiners will undergo what amounts to an apprenticeship, typically lasting two years or so, during which they need to be given the chance to work cases (as many as possible and with as wide a range of examination types – from handwriting to printing to altered documents – as come into the laboratory) while being mentored by an experienced expert.

To be able to do the job effectively, attention to detail, an enquiring mind, a methodical approach to practical problems and 'stickability' are all assets for the would-be expert. But the final product of most examinations in all areas of forensic practice is not 'the conclusion' itself, but rather the report or statement that is given to the investigator and which, ultimately, may end up presented in court as part of the evidence in a case. For this reason, it is also necessary that the practitioner has sufficient skills in writing clearly and concisely in order to describe the pertinent points of their examination for others (non-experts in the field) to understand. All of which can end up with the expert giving oral evidence in person, and this too requires another set of public speaking skills that do not come easily to a lot of people.

Jobs in forensic document examination are becoming fewer in the UK and perhaps in other countries too. This is in part likely to be a reflection of technological changes in that much that used to be done on paper is now done electronically. Nonetheless, there are still plenty of cases requiring the skills of the document examiner.

References

Dyer, A. G., Found, B., & Rogers, D. (2006). Visual attention and expertise for forensic signature analysis. *Journal of Forensic Sciences*, 51(6), 1397–1404. doi:10.1111/j.1556-4029.2006.00269.x ER.

Found, B., & Ganas, J. (2013). The management of domain irrelevant context information in forensic handwriting examination casework. *Science & Justice*, 53(2), 154–158. doi:10.1016/j.scijus.2012.10.004

Kahneman, D. (2011). *Thinking, Fast and Slow*, Allen Lane, London.

Kelly, J. S., & Lindblom, B. S. (2006). In Kelly J. S., Lindblom B. S. (Eds), *Scientific Examination of Questioned Documents* (2nd edition), CRC Press, London.

National Research Council. (2009). *Strengthening Forensic Science in the United States: A Path Forward*. The National Academies Press, Washington DC.

Risinger, D. M., Denbeaux, M. P., & Saks, M. J. (1989). Exorcism of ignorance as a proxy for rational knowledge: The case of handwriting identification 'expertise'. *University of Pennsylvania Law Review*, 137, 731.

2
Handwriting Development and Comparison

2.1 Introduction

Forensic document examiners routinely give evidence relating to disputed authorship of handwriting and signatures (Ellen, 2006). This chapter looks at both the process and the product of handwriting and how it is examined by the forensic expert. The examination of signatures is considered in the next chapter.

Inevitably, the attention of the forensic handwriting expert is focused on the product – that is the handwriting itself – and relatively little attention may be given to the process that caused the handwriting to be created. Having said which, handwriting experts often infer some of the immediate factors affecting the process from the product. For example, the speed of writing may be inferred from its apparent fluency, or the naturalness of the handwriting from letterforms that are typical or otherwise. More distant factors, such as those affecting the development of handwriting in an individual, may be less thought about, but in general terms they are just as important because they underpin and justify the handwriting experts' ability to do their job. For these reasons, it is important to understand why we write the way we do and why we all differ from one another in this complex skill.

2.2 The process of writing

Handwriting is a highly developed skill that we usually start to acquire during early childhood which then develops during subsequent years through

Foundations of Forensic Document Analysis: Theory and Practice, First Edition. Michael Allen.
© 2016 John Wiley & Sons, Ltd. Published 2016 by John Wiley & Sons, Ltd.
Companion Website: www.wiley.com/go/allen/forensicanalysis

adolescence and early adulthood. By early adulthood handwriting has matured into a settled style that will remain largely unchanged for many years until such time as factors that are detrimental to handwriting production start to affect it, such as illness and old age.

Handwriting acquisition is one of many skills that are learned during the early years of life. There are a number of theories that set out to explain general skill acquisition, be it riding a bike, playing the piano or learning to write. These theories have the aim of connecting what we see in skill development in individuals with an understanding of how this correlates with what is happening in the brain. In particular, there is the idea that specific areas of the brain are pre-destined by virtue of their neurological connections to carry out particular functions (for example, see (Fodor, 1983)), suggesting that certain parts of the brain are associated with different sub-elements of the handwriting process (see Box 2.1).

Box 2.1 Brain function in writing

The brain is made up of many different regions that have different functions. The brain is a very complex physiological structure with different types of cells. The nerve cells, or neurons, communicate with one other using various chemical messengers that affect the electrical properties of the neurons. Other types of cell assist with, and may influence, these electrical and chemical processes. The brain is also lateralised with a left half and a right half with some functions occurring on one side rather than the other.

The brain receives information from the body, such as the shape and colour of an animal seen by the eyes. Conversely, the brain can send information to the body, such as when it tells the eyes to track the animal being viewed. The brain can also process the information to determine the type of animal being viewed, its likely movement path and whether or not it poses a threat to the observer.

The brain has compartments associated with the many functions that it controls. Effective movement of the body (motor coordination) is something that is taken for granted, but in young children the fine control of movement is by no means a straightforward task and manipulation of a writing implement at speed requires a great deal more concentration than is needed by a highly practised adult writer.

Various areas of the brain will be associated with the movement needed to produce handwriting. The relevant messages need to be sent from the brain to the muscles controlling wrist, hand and finger movement, for example, to move the pen in the appropriate way to write the letters. The pen movements, some of which may be curved – further complicating matters, require the muscles to function in the correct sequence at the correct time and with the correct amount of movement. The speed of the movement is also important since if the pen moves too quickly it may produce over-large handwriting or too slowly may produce handwriting that is very small. The pen speed is not constant but must accelerate and decelerate to start and finish the pen stroke. These dynamic aspects of handwriting production are coordinated in the relevant brain areas.

Writing also requires material to be written. The sentences and words used and the meanings that they convey to the reader are constructed by other parts of the brain that are concerned with higher levels of thought in the cortex, the main 'thinking' part of the brain. Just as young children have not yet developed fine control of movement, they also have much less developed use of language and vocabulary and this too will impact on the writing process. Specific areas of the brain are associated with language and these must connect with the areas used for movement to link the language and movement elements needed for handwriting.

The capacity of the brain to carry out tasks is limited and this capacity is often called working memory. This means that tasks compete for the working memory available and the more conscious effort and thought that a task requires, the greater the working memory needed. Or put another way, to reduce working memory for a task it is important that it be more automatically carried out. Hence learning *how* to write to the point where it is automatic will free up the working memory to focus on *what* to write.

Much of the knowledge about brain function has been obtained from medical studies in patients who have particular conditions, such as a stroke, leading to loss of function in particular areas of the brain. More recently, imaging technology such as fMRI (functional magnetic resonance imaging) and PET (positron emission tomography) can create detailed images of the brain structure and its functioning.

One of the cornerstones of handwriting analysis is the observation that handwriting varies both for a given writer and between writers. This concept of variability is central to some theories of how psychological processes work (for example see (Siegler, 2002)) and is profoundly distinct from the frequently encountered notion of finding commonality in psychological processes that aim to show underlying factors shared between individuals. Siegler emphasised the need to embrace variability in order to obtain an understanding of the differences that occur in psychological processes, a view shared by Miller (2002) who reviewed the potential gains to be made from studying variability in cognitive processes. Indeed, Z. Yan and Fischer (2002) suggest that careful, detailed examination of variation is not only desirable but crucial for illuminating the dynamic nature of learning and development in individuals.

Their work, based in part on studying the learning of new routines, showed that performance of a task did not show a simple linear improvement with practice over time, but rather periodically suddenly got better and also sometimes worsened depending on various factors that could be a reflection of the task or the person or both – it found variability both within and between participants in the dynamics of their ability to learn.

Specific areas of the brain are involved in handwriting production and these show up on brain scans, as has been demonstrated in many studies. For example, the speed of writing was examined using PET and various areas of the brain cortex were found to be implicated in the control of pen speed (Siebner et al., 2002). The handwriting of skilful and less skilful children has been examined using fMRI, with particular areas of the brain being associated with differences in skill (Richards et al., 2011). Exactly how the various factors involved in handwriting fit together to enable its smooth and efficient production will now be considered.

2.3   Models of writing production

Models of writing production (as opposed to handwriting production) have been dominated by the ideas put forward by Hayes and Flower (Gregg, L.W. & Steinberg, E. R., 1980), who proposed that writing consists first of a planning stage, then a translating phase and finally a reviewing phase. Roughly, these equated to the creation of ideas (the planning phase), their transformation into words which are set down (the translation phase) and finally the review phase (by reading what has been produced) to check that the product is suitable. Thus, often handwriting as an act is the product of a creative process that determines what to write and how it is to be written. If the words are dictated by someone else or are copied then the planning phase does not apply. Changes in the capability of the writer occur as the translation phase improves with greater handwriting skill, changes that occur during childhood and into adolescence. These are reflected in the development of overall writing skill with increasing age (McCutchen, 2000).

The mental resource within which writing (and handwriting or indeed typing) is carried out is referred to as working memory, which is considered to be a mental mechanism for storing and processing information in the short term and thus providing an interface between incoming perceptual inputs, outgoing actions and longer term memory processes (Baddeley, 2003). The concept of working memory is one that implies a limitation on what 'thoughts' can be stored and processed successfully at a given time. Its relevance to handwriting production is that there is potential competition between the needs of the cognitive (what to write) and the motor (how to write) in terms of working memory resource. It follows from this that the more the physical process of handwriting can be automated in a writer, the more this frees up the working memory for the cognitive elements of writing. For this reason, much of the effort in teaching handwriting to children, after the initial phase of learning letterforms, is focused on increasing speed and automaticity thereby minimising the need for working memory to deal with the mechanics of handwriting and allowing greater capacity for the more conceptual elements of writing (Berninger et al., 2010). Such changes have been found to occur in most children where kinematic factors in handwriting were measured and to change significantly with age (Rueckriegel et al., 2008). The handwriting from participants with ages ranging from 6 to 18 was analysed using a digitising pad (see Box 2.2) to measure various parameters of handwriting production. The authors found a significant correlation between the age of the participants and the velocity of writing, automaticity, movement variability and pen pressure. Automaticity was measured by the number of changes of velocity in pen strokes during handwriting production, providing evidence that there are improvements in the motor elements of handwriting as children get older.

Box 2.2 Digitising pads

Digitising pads are devices that record the movements of a specially adapted pen (similar to a computer tablet and stylus) during handwriting. They enable not just the position of the pen to be determined, but also, for example, the speed of pen movement and the pressure used. The data are recorded very fast, typically 200 times per second, so that very detailed measurements can be made of the behaviour of the pen during the writing process. Using the information from such devices, the speed of pen movement can be determined, from which the acceleration and deceleration of the pen can also be computed.

The data obtained using these devices is used in many areas of hand-writing research because it gives objective measurements of handwriting production and data that can be analysed statistically. For example, if some children appear to have problems with their handwriting then use of the digitising pad may show exactly what the problem is in terms of control of movement. Similarly, some adults who suffer loss of handwriting skill due to a particular circumstance (such as the onset of Parkinson's disease) may show difficulties with certain aspects of pen control.

Greater automaticity, greater speed and reduced variability all suggest that older writers are using highly learned processes to generate handwriting movements, while their younger colleagues are still having to think about how to write. This is consistent with developing neurological patterns of movement that are called upon routinely by the writer and that require little conscious input. While changes in the *appearance* of the handwriting cannot be inferred from these kinematic factors alone, these findings show that the process of handwriting changes as children get older.

Handwriting production is usually considered to be largely a linear process in the sense that information is passed sequentially from one stage to the next (as opposed to parallel processing where information is passed from one stage to two or more subsequent stages at the same time). Handwriting is also thought to be a modular process with high-level ideas (what to write) passed down towards the peripheral motor output (the act of writing itself), with certain regions of the brain being associated with different modules of the process, a model which is in keeping with and an extension of the model of writing production described by Hayes and Flower (Gregg, L.W. and Steinberg, E.R., 1980). Van Galen (1991) suggests that the stages are idea creation, leading to concepts, from which come phrases and then their component words, then the graphemes (the mental representation of letters, such as **B**) and their different letterforms (allographs, for example using **b** rather than *ℓ*), which finally lead to the relevant pen stroke movements.

The effective execution of handwriting requires an element of planning to make the process efficient, with the brain forming a motor plan to move the muscles and joints of the hand and wrist and fingers in a coordinated way to make appropriate pen stroke movements (but see also Box 2.3 for other modes of writing production).

Box 2.3 Mouth and foot writing

For the vast majority, writing is executed using the hand. However, some people who, for whatever reason, are not able to use their hands to write can use alternative approaches, most commonly using the foot or the mouth to hold the writing implement. The models of handwriting production might be expected to be similar except that the muscles and joints in the mouth and foot would be the target of the motor planning rather than the hand and wrist.

Some people may be born with a disability that requires them to use other means of writing production, but for others it may be that they learn to write normally and some trauma causes a sudden loss of the normal means of writing production and hence a re-learning period will be required to become efficient at writing in the new way.[1]

Motor planning is determined by the sequence and shape of the letters that are about to be written. This in turn may be based on the recall of appropriate

---

[1] See, for example, http://www.telegraph.co.uk/news/newstopics/howaboutthat/8325437/Chinese -amputee-boy-taught-to-write-with-his-feet.html.

syllable structure for the word (within the constraints of a syllabic language such as English). Kandel et al. (2006) found that syllable structure constrained motor production in writing, with inter-syllable boundaries being associated with a slowing down of pen movement. This suggests that at this level, the syllable (a unit based on the *sound* of the word) plays a part in the dynamic of the writing process. The combinations of letters within syllables, particularly those that occur more frequently, might become learned as a single 'unit' rather than as a sequence of individual letters. In this context, similar movements may produce different outcomes, such as when the letter pair **e-l** and the single letter **d** are written (Figure 2.1). Wing and Nimmo-Smith (1987) found that the kinetics of pen movement when writing e-l are not the same as the kinetics when writing d, even though the pen path is similar in both instances. This suggests that there is an element of learned, anticipatory context-dependent production in the writing process, consistent with the syllabic element of word construction. In other words, once we know what we are about to write, the letter groupings that make up the syllables of the about to be written words 'queue up' as part of the planning process, awaiting their production on the page as each set of movements in sequence turns the thought into handwritten actions.

The movements themselves are, in a skilled writer, rapid and highly time-coordinated (Longstaff & Heath, 2003). The pen movements have a very tightly controlled dynamic component that ensures that movement changes occur in the right sequence and at an appropriate velocity, without which pen strokes might be of inappropriate size or might not be correctly constructed in relation to one another. The rapidity shows that the movements are planned and held in readiness to be executed in a time-sequenced manner, with a series of overlapping discrete movements generating a smooth continual movement (Morasso et al., 1983).

Handwriting movements are constrained by the anatomy and neurological capability of the writer's arm, wrist, hand and finger movements as a result of which some pen movements are preferred to others as they are more readily executed (Thomassen et al., 1991). The smoothness and consistency of movement of arm joints and muscles improves during childhood and is often of an adult standard at the age of about 11 or 12 (Chiappedi et al., 2012) – an age at which handwriting skills are still being perfected.

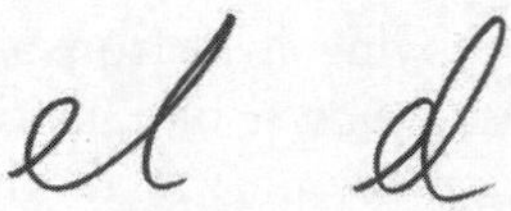

Figure 2.1 A similar pen path is used for writing the letter **d** and the letter pair **el**.

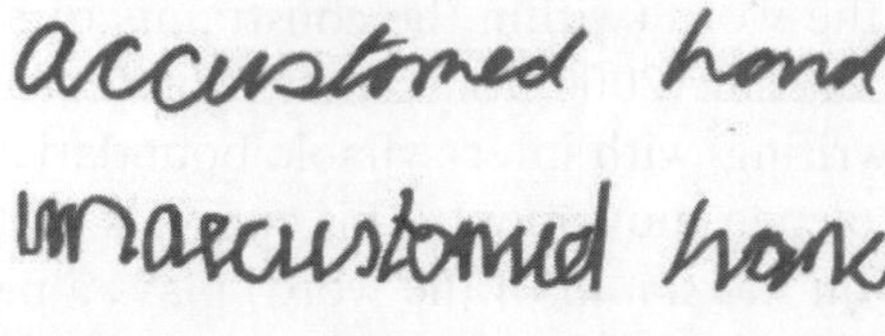

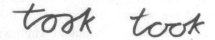

Figure 2.2   Handwriting from same person using accustomed and unaccustomed hand.

Figure 2.3   Handwriting with clockwise and right to left t-crossbar (left-hand example) and anticlockwise and left to right t-crossbar (right-hand example).

Handedness in handwriting production is another consideration and is of particular interest to the forensic expert. This is because if the handedness of the writer of a piece of handwriting can be determined this may provide important evidence of authorship, since for many people writing with the unaccustomed hand is difficult, leading to poor fluency (Figure 2.2). Evidence relating to handedness may be available from the pen movements made (Figure 2.3), since left-handed writers often prefer clockwise and right-to-left movements due to the biomechanics of the muscles and joints that are in mirror image to those of right-handed writers, who generally prefer to use anti-clockwise and left-to-right movements (Meulenbroek & Van Galen, 1989). It is perhaps noteworthy that not all writing systems follow the same pattern of left-to-right alphabetic construction. For example, Arabic is also alphabetic but written right to left, and other writing systems do not use alphabets at all (see Box 2.4).

Box 2.4 Non-Roman writing scripts

The subject of language structure and its written form is very complex with many variations between different systems. However, some general rules do apply to most of them. The historical origins of writing systems go back thousands of years and the earliest systems used drawings of objects as opposed to words as we understand them today. However, over hundreds of years, the need to write down more complex ideas that could not readily be drawn led to changes, moving away from a drawing to more abstract writing systems. For example, a *picture* of a hand 🖐 may be readily understood without any learning on the part of the reader, whereas the *word* 'hand' written down requires the reader to have learned its meaning as the letters **h-a-n-d** have no connection to the idea of a hand.

English is written in the Roman script as are many other languages. Words are composed of sequences of individual, alphabetic letters, a system of writing that is shared with other writing systems such as Cyrillic (used in the Slav countries such as Russia and Serbia) and Greek. These systems also share the idea of capital letterforms. Arabic is also alphabetic but it is written right to left and it does not contain any capital letters. Alphabetic systems relate the individual letters (and their combinations) to the sound that they make when spoken, although there are many obvious exceptions to this general rule.

In logographic writing systems, a grapheme (written character) represents a whole word and there is no direct relationship between the written symbol and the sound of the word it represents. Examples include Chinese and Japanese.

The effect of losing the use of the dominant hand (for most people this is the right hand) has been studied clinically, but it is difficult to generalise over what the impact will be on a given writer as each case is different (Yancosek & Mullineaux, 2011), albeit many writers are able to write reasonably well with subsequent retraining using the unaccustomed hand if given enough practice (Walker & Henneberg, 2007).

When examining a piece of handwriting, the direction of pen stroke can often be determined by a careful examination of the ink line. In particular, the presence of striations within a ballpoint pen ink line can show the direction of travel of the pen, with striations going from the inside to the outside of a curved pen stroke even if the degree of curvature is slight (see Section 2.8.2). Inferring the handedness of a writer should always be done with caution as a small minority of writers can use both hands equally well and not all writers use all of the handwriting traits associated with left- or right-handed writing.

The models that describe the process of handwriting production show just what a neurologically complex process it is and provide clear evidence for the scope of variability in handwriting both between different writers and within the writing of the same person. A consideration of the many external factors that influence the learning of handwriting will now show additional forces that affect the development of handwriting within an individual from childhood through adolescence and into adulthood.

2.4 The learning of handwriting in young children

Learning to write is regarded as one of the most important skills that a child can acquire in early school years. Given the opportunity, children as young as 12 months old like to make marks on paper with writing implements. The use of a writing/drawing implement begins in young children when they can pick it up and manipulate it in such a way as to make a mark on a substrate (usually paper). The ability to make marks and their associated meanings, which in time come to be attributed to such marks, are the embryonic stages of drawing (Kellogg, 1969). Kellogg found that the early scribblings of young children can be deconstructed into a number of common elements consisting of various orientations of lines, circular movements, zigzags and other similar movements. These movements are in essence those which are to be found in handwriting later on in a child's development.

One thing that is striking about the process of learning to draw is the use of repeated sets of movements by the child to replicate in a formulaic manner frequently drawn images (Hollis & Low, 2005). Rather than re-invent a new series of pen strokes to draw a house or a face, the young child first learns a sequence of strokes needed to produce a satisfactory image and then uses the same set of movements each time they draw that item. Of course, because of the inherent complexity of the motor and cognitive elements involved in drawing, no two drawings are absolutely identical; instead, they will show variation from one to another. Rueckriegel et al. (2008) showed that the automaticity of *both* drawing and writing movements increased as children got older, providing additional evidence for a maturation process in the motor components of both handwriting and drawing.

The idea that the ability to draw and the ability to write are connected has been widely investigated. Those who are proficient at drawing are also likely to be proficient at producing handwriting, as found by Bonoti et al. (2005). They showed a correlation between handwriting and drawing skills in 182 children aged 8–12 years old, scoring handwriting in terms of placement, conforming to taught styles and size and scoring drawings, such as a man or a house, to set descriptors of how they were drawn.

A number of general aspects of development in younger children's handwriting have been studied, including legibility, speed and size (Blote & Hamstra-Bletz, 1991; Graham et al., 1998; Rueckriegel et al., 2008). Handwriting speed and legibility in children aged 6–15 was studied and were both found to improve year on year, although the rate of change varied with, for example, those aged 6–10 improving more rapidly than those in the next few years (Graham et al., 1998). Graham et al. also found that legibility generally improved with age, but that again the rate of change was not even, with little improvement in the younger years and greater improvements in later years. Handwriting size tends to start larger in those learning to write, decreases in size over the next few years and thereafter some children start to write larger again (Blote & Hamstra-Bletz, 1991).

Developmental processes of handwriting change in older children attract relatively little attention in the literature (Weintraub et al., 2007). However, neurological problems in children during these formative years can lead to a range of problems in later years in terms of the legibility and correctness of the handwriting formation and its speed of execution (van Hoorn et al., 2010a). One of the reasons why handwriting attracts little attention in the later phases of development is that handwriting ability is no longer perceived as being a constraining factor on learning for most children and older children are thought to be less amenable to instruction in the case of any dysfunction. This may be a short-sighted view, however, as a child's handwriting is unlikely to improve on its own but rather requires help, and later academic performance may indeed be influenced by the ability to execute handwriting effectively (Feder & Majnemer, 2007).

The way in which the writing implement is held at the paper surface is one of the last links between the internal (biological) processes of handwriting production and its physical manifestation on the paper. Tseng (1998), for example, identifies over a dozen pencil grips in children in the 3–6 year old age range, although the number of grips used falls off with increased age as inappropriate grips are discarded by those who tried them. This is echoed by the findings of Schneck and Henderson (1990) who identify ten grips that are associated with different levels of development in children, with different grips sometimes used for different tasks, such as writing and colouring in, and with gender differences between preferred grips. Nevertheless, some children will find particular grips more comfortable than others and this is likely to be in part determined by the suppleness of their finger and wrist joints (Summers, 2001) and hence the amount of pen control that a particular grip gives the child (Burton & Dancisak, 2000). Changes in pen grip are almost bound to lead to increased variation of the handwriting since this will influence the overall fine motor movement. Indeed, the movements of muscle sets involved in handwriting have been found to be less variable in older children who can write more quickly than younger children (Naider-Steinhart & Katz-Leurer, 2007).

A significant proportion of children will have some difficulty learning to write (Hoy, et al., 2011) and a variety of techniques is used in an attempt to improve a child's handwriting, focusing often on general visual and motor integration and fine control skills (Feder & Majnemer, 2007). The techniques used will also vary depending on the root cause of the problems, such as those attributable to various medical conditions, but the main criterion for referral is generally simply the teacher finding it difficult to read the child's handwriting (Hammerschmidt & Sudsawad, 2004). A method for measuring handwriting capability is central to such techniques and a number have been devised; they are summarised in Box 2.5.

The process of learning to write, therefore, contains many factors that have the potential to affect a child's handwriting. The earliest experiences of acquiring the skill of handwriting are now passed on into the middle school years of adolescence, where yet more changes will occur.

Box 2.5 Assessing handwriting in children

A variety of tests aimed at assessing handwriting in children have been proposed. Their purpose has generally been either to show changes in handwriting ability with age or to provide an objective measure when individual writers are having problems learning to write. Some of these are noted here with a view to illustrating the kinds of parameters of handwriting that are assessed in this context.

The BHK (*Beknopte beoordelingsmethode voor kinderhandschriften*) test was devised as a means of assessing handwriting quality in children who have difficulty in producing handwriting (dysgraphia). The original paper is in Dutch, but the procedures are summarised elsewhere (for example, Kaiser et al., 2009) and involve a handwriting task requiring the copying of a text in five minutes or the first five lines, whichever is the greater amount, albeit only the first five lines are scored in any event. The text becomes increasingly complex and at the same time each successive paragraph is reproduced in a smaller font. The child does this task without having had the opportunity to see the text and the handwriting is done on unlined paper. Scoring of the handwriting is based on a variety of features that assess deviations from the taught style according to 13 criteria; letter size, left margin widening, poor word alignment, insufficient word spacing, acute turns in connecting letters or too long joining, irregularities in joining strokes, collision of letters, inconsistent letter size, incorrect relative height of letters, letter distortion, ambiguous letterforms, correction of letterforms, and unsteady writing trace.

A number of other schemes have been devised to assess handwriting in children including:

- the Minnesota Handwriting Assessment (Reisman, J. (1999) London, UK, Harcourt Assessment);

- the Test of Legible Handwriting (TOLH), which has been used by various researchers (for example, Graham et al., 2006);

- the Scale of Children's Readiness In PrinTing (SCRIPT) has been developed and used (for example, Marr et al., 2001);

- the Evaluation Tool of Children's Handwriting (ETCH), which was developed by Amundson and has been used by a number of authors (for example, Koziatek & Powell, 2002); and

- the Children's Handwriting Evaluation Scale (CHES) devised by Phelps et al. (1985).

2.5 Handwriting in the adolescent: the origins of individuality

A person's handwriting can change at any time, but generally from early adulthood through to early old age a person's handwriting is fairly stable. However, the handwriting of adolescents and those entering old age is more likely to change over time. In the former group this is because the handwriting has not yet fully developed and in the latter it is because there may be a general skill deterioration associated with old age.

Little has been published about handwriting development as it occurs in adolescents, spanning the years from about the age of 10 to late teens. By the time most writers reach the age of about 10 they have acquired a reasonable degree of fluency and speed in the production of handwriting (Weintraub et al., 2007). However, that is not to say that in these writers the developmental process stops; far from it, for once the essential elements of the skill of handwriting have been mastered, it is then possible for the writer to manipulate it to their own ends, rather like learning the basics of tennis strokes and then developing and perfecting them to fit best with your own physical capabilities. For handwriting, development during adolescence may be in terms of general features, such as the speed and legibility of the handwriting (Graham et al., 1998), or in more specific details of the letterforms used, introducing shapes and forms of letters that were not taught them at all but adopting new features for any one of a variety of reasons – from peer compliance to parental guidance (Sassoon, 1990).

It is during the adolescent years that the handwriting of an individual goes through some of its most transformative stages, becoming, on the one hand, more consistent and, on the other hand, more individual. Allen (2011) found that the handwriting of children becomes increasingly consistent with age and at the same time also becomes more differentiated from their peers. This was shown by taking a series of letterforms and determining how their use changed over time in children aged 5–18. Within-writer variability was greatest in children aged about 10 or 11 years old suggesting a period of experimentation and change, whereas individualisation was greatest in the older children, as shown by a strong tendency for samples of handwriting of a given individual to be similar one to another but different from that of his or her peers.

It is obvious that most adults' handwriting is markedly different from that taught to them as children not just in terms of general appearance and skill but also when considering specific letterforms. Changes to handwriting over the years of adolescence are largely gradual but can occasionally be more sudden, especially when a writer intentionally incorporates new features into their writing during periods of experimentation. The additional effect of striving for increased speed will also drive some of these changes as the writer becomes not only quicker but adopts a handwriting style that is more efficient in terms of pen movement, letter joining and other relevant dynamic factors. Despite this, some writers will produce handwriting of a particular style that is not so dynamically efficient, sacrificing speed for appearance. The many factors impacting upon the handwriting of an individual are particularly likely to have an effect at this time, when the basic skill of handwriting has been acquired but before it has been fully developed into a mature personal style. Given the complexity of the effects of these factors on one another, it is not surprising that at the end of the period of adolescence, each individual child's handwriting has become more distinctively their own.

The handwriting of adolescents causes some difficulties for the forensic expert since its immaturity, variability and any imitative components from within the taught or peer groups can all have short-term impacts on its appearance (Cusack & Hargett, 1989). These factors must be considered carefully when interpreting the significance of observations in casework, and there is a particular need to ensure that any specimens of handwriting are as contemporary as practicable with the handwriting in question so as to minimise differences that can occur over short time periods. This is usually less critical when considering the handwriting of adults, which will be considered next.

2.6   Mature handwriting of the adult

In Sections 2.4 and 2.5 the importance of learning and developing handwriting was emphasised in relation to its impact on how people end up writing as adults. The teaching of handwriting has changed over time and varies from place to place. This leads to general style differences and also to some character-specific variations being found in the writings from those taught in different places and at different times. In many countries, an elaborate version of handwriting was traditionally taught, such as copperplate. Whilst this may have been elegant and aesthetically appealing, over time simpler styles were considered more appropriate in terms of the ease with which children could learn to write. These educational and cultural influences will lead to an increase in variation between writers who are taught different so-called copybook styles.

Some differences are attributable to the prevailing method of teaching at a particular time in a particular country. A number of systems are outlined in the book by Huber and Headrick (1999: chapter 8) showing styles of handwriting from a number of countries. For example the following would be regarded as unusual by someone taught to write in the UK (Figure 2.4): the letter **W** constructed from four separate pen strokes – this is commonplace in many taught to write in West Africa; the use of the capital form of the letter **R** in lower case writing is a habit found commonly in the writing of those taught in Ireland; the numeral 7 written with a crossbar is widely regarded as a European affectation although increasingly common in the UK; the number 9 written with a

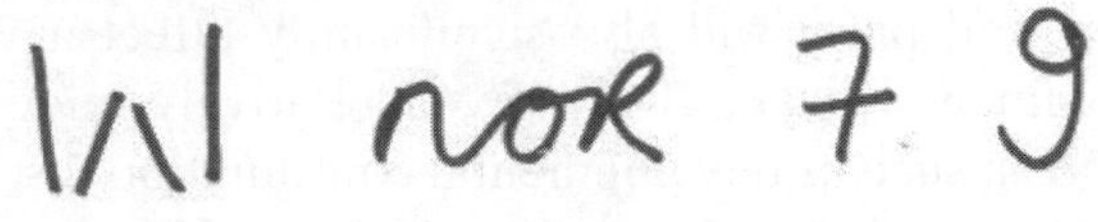

Figure 2.4   Examples of national handwriting characteristics (see text).

markedly curved tail and often using two pen strokes is common in eastern Europe (Turnbull et al., 2010).

Such features are not necessarily universal, but they do tend to occur with greater frequency in some groups than others and hence provide another source for between-writer variation in a multi-cultural society.

The effects of these cultural influences are shown by the findings of Cheng et al. (2005) when examining the writings of three culturally distinct groups, namely Chinese, Indian (writing Tamil) and Malay (writing Arabic) people in Singapore, learning to write English as a second language. These three handwriting systems have very different appearances and this was reflected in the romanised English written by individuals from these different backgrounds. For example, the stress on straight lines in Chinese, the formation of dots in Arabic and the curvature of the strokes in Tamil were reflected in the writing in English.

As far as the handwriting expert is concerned, therefore, it is important to be aware of changes in taught handwriting styles over time and in different places and to make any necessary enquiries when examining handwriting that shows such influences. There would then be a need for information to be supplied about the nationality and age of those providing handwriting specimens so that the expert can interpret the findings giving appropriate significance to the features present.

2.7   The deterioration of handwriting skill

A variety of factors can lead to deterioration in handwriting including various medical conditions, the effects of alcohol and some drugs that affect the central nervous system, as well as increasing old age. Generally, these factors impact on either the cognitive or the motor aspects of handwriting production, disrupting at some point the pathway from thought to movement of the hand and fingers. Underlying these conditions is brain function, which is required for handwriting production (see Box 2.1).

While illness might generally be thought a factor in the handwriting of adults and, more specifically, the elderly, in fact there are a number of medical conditions that can affect handwriting in young people. Children and adolescents with autism spectrum disorder (ASD) are likely to show poorly constructed letterforms associated with reduced motor control (Fuentes et al., 2010). Cerebral palsy will also significantly affect a young person's handwriting (Bumin & Kavak, 2010). Even relatively minor neurological dysfunctions (MND), such as developmental coordination disorder, can have an impact on the handwriting of young people (van Hoorn et al., 2010b) in terms of legibility, speed and appropriate formation.

Handwriting errors that occur as a result of brain damage, typically after a lesion caused by a stroke, are of a number of kinds and reflect the areas of the brain affected and their role in the processing of information from cognitive to motor output. Errors can occur at the level of allograph choice, in which the style and case of the letters are determined, and damage to this process would be expected to lead, for example, to an inappropriate mixing of upper and lower case letters (Debastiani & Barry, 1989). Once the style and case are chosen the next stage is to adopt the appropriate set of movements to write the letter and errors at this point will lead to substitution of correctly formed but incorrect letters (Destreri et al., 2000). A lesion that disrupts the motor pattern will produce handwriting that is poorly formed so that it tends towards an illegible scribble (Margolin & Wing, 1983). Other medical conditions can cause very small writing, known as micrographia, including loss of blood flow to certain parts of the brain, a condition which can be reversible (Perrin et al., 2005).

Micrographia is most often associated with patients with Parkinson's disease. Indeed, micrographia is a well-established clinical indicator of Parkinson's disease with about three-quarters of patients showing it as a symptom (Bryant et al., 2010). Bryant and colleagues show that it may be possible to at least partially overcome micrographia using grid lines to help the writer to adjust letter size. Medical intervention, such as levodopa prescribed to alleviate the symptoms of Parkinson's, may reduce the micrographia (Tucha et al., 2006a) and subsequent stopping of the medication leads to a worsening of the effects on handwriting production. The effects of levodopa on handwriting performance may be noticeable just minutes or hours after being administered (Poluha et al., 1998).

Patients with multiple sclerosis do not normally have difficulty writing but have a tendency to write more slowly (Rosenblum & Weiss, 2010). This will be reflected in the apparent fluency of the handwriting as indicated by the evidence of pen speed across the paper.

A more general deterioration of writing capability is commonly found in patients with Alzheimer's disease or associated mild cognitive impairment with slower, less smooth and less consistent handwriting (Yan et al., 2008), with both the content (such as misspellings and semantic substitutions) and its motor execution being affected, with the former often occurring before the latter as the disease progressively worsens (Croisile, 1999).

Because certain medical conditions are manifested in handwriting, it may be possible to tentatively diagnose such conditions from an assessment of a person's handwriting. For example the handwriting errors that typically occur in those with Alzheimer's may be used (even posthumously) to ascertain a person's capacity to understand, for example, a document signed by them (Balestrino et al., 2012). Indeed, there is a link between handwriting and general cognitive dysfunction in the elderly in terms of handwriting ability (Ericsson et al., 1996), with deterioration of the signature being more resistant to such effects than general handwriting.

Not all medical conditions that impact on handwriting necessarily have an obvious neurological cause. For example, one study has shown that cirrhosis of the liver can affect a person's handwriting, albeit the mechanism linking them has not been established (Mechtcheriakov et al., 2006). Conditions that are more in the domain of psychiatry, such as obsessive compulsive disorder (OCD), have also been shown to have some subtle motor effects that are then transmitted to handwriting leading to slower, less well-automated handwriting (Mavrogiorgou et al., 2001).

The automatic nature of skilful handwriting is such that it might be expected that blindness, particularly if its onset occurred after the skill had been acquired, will affect the appearance of handwriting. However, there is a need for visual feedback in the process of handwriting and the absence of this will cause errors to occur (Arter et al., 1996).

The elderly are often some of the most vulnerable in society and therefore the target of criminal activity. For this reason the handwriting capabilities of the elderly need to be understood by the handwriting expert in order to be able to interpret findings in cases involving old people.

Elderly, but otherwise healthy, people do not generally have a great need to write extensively but rather tend to make infrequent, short jotting-type notes (van Drempt et al., 2011). In such circumstances, it is not surprising that in the absence of regular use of the skill the authors found that handwriting was particularly variable in terms of parameters such as baseline position, inter-word spacing and slope. Handwriting speed gets slower as people get older beyond the age of about 65 (Burger & McCluskey, 2011) and in older people the task and even the type of writing implement used can affect handwriting speed.

In only a few instances has the forensic significance of these medical factors been considered by handwriting experts. For example, the effects of Parkinson's disease (Walton, 1997) and of recent blindness (Masson, 1988) have been reported. However, only broad categories of effects can be reported due to the variable responses of people to medical impacts on their handwriting, making it difficult to generalise from one case to another.

In forensic casework, the most frequently encountered intoxicant is alcohol. The effects of alcohol on handwriting have been studied and often show a diminution in the control of pen movement rather than specific errors in handwriting production. A variety of spatial measures including word length, heights of letters, heights of ascenders (such as the left side of a letter **h**) and descenders (such as the tail of the letter **y**), and the spacing between words have been shown to be significantly affected by alcohol (Asicioglu & Turan, 2003). The reasons for the effects of alcohol on motor functions shown in handwriting are not fully understood but they are similar to the effects of cerebellar dysfunction in the brain (Phillips et al., 2009).

The forensic impact of alcohol on handwriting has been considered (Beck, 1985; Galbraith, 1986) but as with the effects of medical conditions, intoxicants have differing effects or similar effects of differing degrees from one person to another, particularly depending on their tolerance of alcohol.

The effects of caffeine have been reported (Dhawn, et al., 1969; Tucha et al., 2006b). Dhawn and colleagues also report on the impact of methamphetamine, chlorpromazine and phenobarbitone in terms of time taken to write, spacing and size of letterforms. Caffeine and methamphetamine are stimulants and lead to faster handwriting, whereas chlorpromazine and phenobarbitone are depressants and slow handwriting. Tucha and colleagues found that caffeine produced faster handwriting with smoother acceleration and deceleration of the pen as measured using a handwriting digitising tablet. These effects were dose related, so the more caffeine taken the greater the effect.

In another study, Tucha and Lange explored the effects of nicotine on handwriting (Tucha & Lange, 2004) and found increased velocity and greater fluency in handwriting production in both smokers and non-smokers with nicotine intake.

There is very little information in the literature about the forensic effects of drugs on handwriting. Commonly encountered drugs, such as caffeine and nicotine, are likely to have marginal effects on letterform but may alter writing speed to some degree. Other drugs that have greater effects on the relevant neurological pathways may have more profound effects on handwriting, especially when they are prescribed to improve an underlying medical condition. Nonetheless, handwriting experts need to be aware of the possibility that these various factors might impact on a person's handwriting.

2.8   The forensic analysis of handwriting

Up to this point in the chapter, the focus has been on the *process* of handwriting. Now the *product* of handwriting will be considered in detail since it is this that the forensic handwriting expert will examine in the real world of casework.

The forensic handwriting expert may be asked to examine all kinds of cases ranging from relatively minor fraud involving small amounts of money through to murder and terrorism. Casework inevitably involves examining material that is constrained by practical considerations. For example, the amount of questioned handwriting in dispute is usually a given, be it an anonymous note, a telephone number scribbled down hurriedly or a death threat. However, an investigator may be able to exert some degree of control over the obtaining of samples of specimen handwriting of known authorship to compare with the questioned handwriting. Requesting specimen samples from a writer provides an opportunity to get as much as is reasonable to expect, or a search of premises may provide other samples. But in reality, the handwriting expert will only have a relatively small amount of handwriting (in comparison to the whole handwritten output of an individual) to examine; typically a handful of questioned documents and a few samples of specimen handwriting – although some cases may be much larger and some even more restricted in terms of available evidence.

The vast majority of cases involving a forensic handwriting examination are centred on a comparison between the disputed handwriting and samples of specimen handwriting from one or more people who are suspected of having produced the handwriting in question. (The forensic examination of handwriting to identify authorship should not be confused with examinations that aim to identify the personality of the writer, often referred to as graphology.)

Of course, each case is unique, but there are a number of steps involved in a forensic handwriting examination that form an appropriate procedure to ensure it is carried out properly. English uses a number of general styles of handwriting that are usually called script (small unjoined letters), cursive (joined letters) and block capitals. Small letters are usually referred to as lower case and capital letters as upper case. Block capital letters are generally dissimilar in form from the letters used in script and cursive handwriting and they cannot be effectively compared. Likewise, the act of joining letters can have an impact on their appearance and so comparing script with cursive handwriting is not ideal. Many writers mix the styles of handwriting that they use. Even skilled writers may join some letters and not others, and some writers may mix upper and lower case letters. As far as the handwriting expert is concerned, the key point is that a comparison can best be done between letterforms that are comparable, usually called a like-with-like comparison. If a case is submitted in which the styles of handwriting to be compared differ, then there needs to be some dialogue between the expert and those submitting the case to try and improve the basis of the examination.

2.8.1 Specimen handwriting

There are two kinds of specimen handwriting that can be obtained in casework. The first is known as a request specimen, since it involves the investigator asking a person to provide a sample of handwriting. The details are typically dictated to the person supplying the handwriting sample and, depending on their cooperativeness, the aim of the investigator is to obtain a reasonable amount of handwriting. The amount will in part be determined by the case. For example, if there is only a single jotted telephone number in question, then obtaining perhaps 10 or 12 repeated versions of that phone number in a specimen is likely to be adequate. But if the questioned handwriting consists of many pages of handwriting, obtaining even one version as a specimen may be too much to expect.

As has been noted above, the process of handwriting is most natural when it is done quickly and with the minimum of conscious input. A specimen of writing written in such a way should be a reasonable sample of a person's handwriting. However, if the writer deliberately disrupts their normal handwriting by consciously trying to alter their handwriting, in other words disguising it, then obtaining such a specimen may not yield a satisfactorily representative sample of their handwriting. To overcome this, it may be necessary for the investigator to try to delay or distract the writer in order to take their focus away from the act of disguising their handwriting and causing them to write more naturally.

If a person is not cooperative in providing a specimen of handwriting at request, it may be possible to obtain a non-request sample of writing from their everyday lives, such as address books, letters, forms or diaries. The handwriting on such documents can generally be assumed to have been written naturally (or at least without intentional disguise), although the circumstances of writing can vary from writing carefully at a table to scribbling something down while standing, for example. A non-request specimen, therefore, has the advantage that it is likely to be naturally written. However, it has the disadvantage that there is no control over its content, so if the questioned handwriting is in cursive handwriting and an address book is supplied containing entries in block capitals and numerals, the specimen may well be naturally written but also largely irrelevant. In addition, there is always a concern over who in fact wrote a non-request specimen and, related to that, whether all of the handwriting is by one person or whether more than one person has written it.

If both request and non-request specimens of handwriting are available, this is often the ideal situation since the former can be controlled to ensure that relevant details are present and the latter should at least be natural and show the normal handwriting skill of the person concerned. In addition, if there is a concern that the requested handwriting is not natural, this can often be confirmed or refuted by checking it against the non-request sample.

The quality of the specimen handwriting obtained is a crucial factor in determining whether a handwriting expert can reach a conclusion over the authorship of a piece of questioned handwriting. If the specimen supplied by an investigator is inadequate for one reason or another, the expert must take this into account and consider the option of asking for more samples before committing themselves to any opinion.

Handwriting undergoes relatively little change during adulthood, but in adolescence and as writers move towards old age and its associated medical conditions, another factor comes into play when considering specimen hand-writing, namely time. If a questioned document was written when someone was in their late 80s and suffering from Parkinson's disease, then a diary writ-ten by them when they were in their 50s may well be of little use. Likewise, a specimen of handwriting from a person aged 16 may not be ideal when com-pared to a questioned note written when they were 13, since their handwriting may well have still been developing during that time. Obtaining contemporary specimens may therefore be very important depending on the case, and again a dialogue between the expert and the investigator may assist.

The writing implement of choice for handwriting specimens is usually the ballpoint pen, but it must be borne in mind that the implement used can affect the handwriting and this may be a factor that the expert needs to consider when assessing the evidence in a case. For this reason, it is necessary to briefly consider writing implements and what influence they may have on a person's handwriting. (A more detailed review of ink examination can be found in Chapter 6.)

2.8.2 Writing implements

In general, the choice of writing implement (or at least conventional writ-ing implements) does not affect the process of writing but it might affect the appearance or the fluency of the writing (Mathyer, 1969). The use of uncon-ventional implements such as a paint brush may well affect the structure of the handwriting. Nonetheless, by far the most commonly encountered writing implement is the ballpoint pen. The viscous ink is held in a reservoir behind a rotating ball bearing (Figure 2.5). Rotation of the ball causes ink to coat the

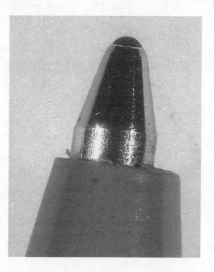

Figure 2.5 The tip of a ballpoint pen (x8 approx.).

ball and be deposited on the paper. Ballpoint pen lines tend to be impressed into the surface of the paper, the extent of which is partly determined by the pressure applied to the pen by the writer. The ink is oil-based and often has a lustrous, thick appearance when viewed under magnification. The deposit of ink may sometimes be uneven, with excess ink occasionally being deposited to form so-called goops. If the pen is unused and the ball is open to the air, the ink may dry on the ball such that when next used this dry ink is lost, producing an inkless start to the pen stroke. Most importantly, many, but not all, ballpoint pens produce striation lines within the ink line. These have the property of indicating the direction of the pen stroke in curved ink lines, with the striation going from the inside to the outside of the line in the direction of motion (Figure 2.6). This may yield important information about the pen movement – for example whether a letter **O** is written clockwise or anticlockwise. It is because of this kind of information that the ballpoint pen is the implement of choice when obtaining handwriting samples at request.

Other pens use a hard rotating ball but with different ink formulations. For example, gel pens use inks that are water-based. Other pens use nibs that are fibrous, such as felt tip pens (Figure 2.7). Some felt tip pens have relatively narrow nibs, but some are much wider – for example, marker pens – and the broad nib makes normal handwriting movements more difficult. Handwriting produced with such writing implements may be structurally different to that produced with more conventional writing implements.

Traditionally, the fountain pen was the implement of choice, but such pens are less and less encountered. They too use water-based ink and the ink line

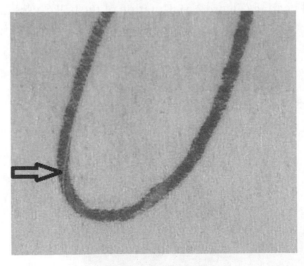

Figure 2.6 Striation lines in a ballpoint pen ink line (x10 approx.). *(See insert for colour representation of the figure.)*

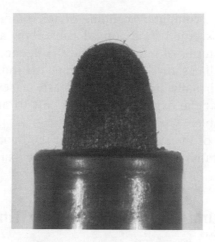

Figure 2.7 A felt tip pen nib (x8 approx.).

is often uneven along the edges. Pencils are occasionally used, typically producing a readily recognisable grey writing line.

Casework can involve handwriting produced with all manner of things ranging from paintbrushes to marks scratched onto wooden surfaces to lipstick. Such unconventional implements inevitably inhibit the normal, natural handwriting movements of the writer and due consideration of this must be given when assessing findings. In addition, the posture of the writer in such cases is also often unusual, such as standing up writing on a vertical surface or bending down writing on a flat surface at ground level. Again, such postural changes can require handwriting movements using unfamiliar joints and muscles and may impact on the handwritten product.

2.8.3 Pre-examination review

Before starting a full case examination, the expert should make sure that the material submitted is suitable given the question that has been asked by the investigator. If the material is not suitable, then the investigator should be contacted with a view to establishing whether there is a realistic prospect of improving matters. As noted above, the questioned and specimen handwritings must be comparable and the specimens must be as relevant as possible. However, there are often other preliminary considerations.

One of the most common problems is poor quality copy documents. Although most handwriting is in original form at some point (an exception might be signatures produced using a stylus on a touch sensitive pad as used by some delivery services, for example), some cases involve the examination of copy documents, that is documents that have been produced by photocopying, faxing, computer scanning or microfilming. The amount of detail that can be discerned from copy documents is always less than that from the original in terms of letterform and the fluency of the handwriting. A copy document that shows the handwriting so indistinctly as to make examination of it virtually impossible is clearly a severe limitation to a comparison such that the expert may feel it best to at least seek a better quality copy if available.

If after a preview of the submitted material the handwriting expert feels that a meaningful examination is possible, then the examination proper can commence.

2.8.4   The natural variation of handwriting

The forensic examination of handwriting is a painstaking process that requires a lot of patience on the part of the expert, an eye for detail and a comprehensive approach together with an unbiased, open mind as to the outcome. There are many sources of information in a piece of handwriting that help inform the expert about whether or not a questioned document was written by a particular person. Central to this assessment is the idea of the natural variation that is to be found in handwriting.

Variation in handwriting is its most important property and yet the one that causes the most problems. As was shown in earlier sections of this chapter, there is considerable scope for handwriting to vary both between different writers and within the handwritten output of the same person, attributable to the highly complex cognitive and motor processes involved. However, this does not mean that handwriting can vary infinitely – far from it. The automatic nature of handwriting in a skilled writer ensures that the writer generally produces letterforms that are similar but not identical from one occasion to another. In another sense handwriting is also constrained by the need for it to be readable, so there are conventional letterforms that are recognisable as conforming to expectations: a letter **A** must at least look like a letter **A**, irrespective of how it is constructed.

But in casework a forensic handwriting expert is confronted with relatively small amounts of handwriting to examine. Even with small amounts of handwriting, research has shown the scope for between-writer variability in, for example, English (Srihari et al., 2002) and Japanese (Ueda et al., 2009).

The variations to be found in handwriting generally occur along a number of dimensions. It is not necessary or possible to catalogue these letter by letter. Instead, an indication is given here of the *kinds* of feature that must be considered when analysing variation in handwriting. In addition, describing handwriting features using words alone is often awkward and hence diagrams are included unless the appearance of the letterform is very obvious from the description given.

Letter construction has a number of different components. For example, the letter **B** can be written in one continuous movement or as two separate pen strokes, or the letter **E** written as a semi-circle with a second, central horizontal stroke or written as an L-shape with two further strokes (see Figure 2.8a).

Characters of similar construction can themselves vary in the sequence of pen movements used to write them. Continuing with the letter **E**, the L-shape can be followed by the top stroke then finally the middle stroke or the middle stroke then the top stroke (Figure 2.8b). Similarly, the top stroke of the letter **T** may be written either before or after the down stroke (Figure 2.8c).

The direction of pen movement may vary and this can sometimes be determined, for example by examining pen striations (see Section 2.8.2). Some write their letter **O** in a clockwise direction (usually, but not always, left-handed writers), others write it anti-clockwise (most right-handed writers and also a significant proportion of left-handed writers) – see Figure 2.3 earlier in the chapter.

The direction of pen movement when writing the numeral 8 may vary, together with the point of initiation. The most common is to commence at the top right and move anticlockwise, the pen finally returning to the top right from the bottom left. But some writers begin at top left and may head anti-clockwise or clockwise, and yet other writers start at bottom left (Figure 2.8d).

Most curved letters, such as the letter **S**, tend to be written starting at the top and finishing at the bottom. However, in a small minority of writers, the letter is begun at the bottom of the letter (Figure 2.8e).

As well as variation in curved movements, writers vary in the horizontal and vertical directions too. For example, some writers write the A-crossbar from left to right and others in the reverse direction. The initiation of many letters, such as **M** or **N**, with a down stroke is frequently encountered, but some writers omit the down stroke and commence with an up stroke (Figure 2.8f).

The proportions of written characters can vary both within themselves and also between various characters, although proportionality is usually

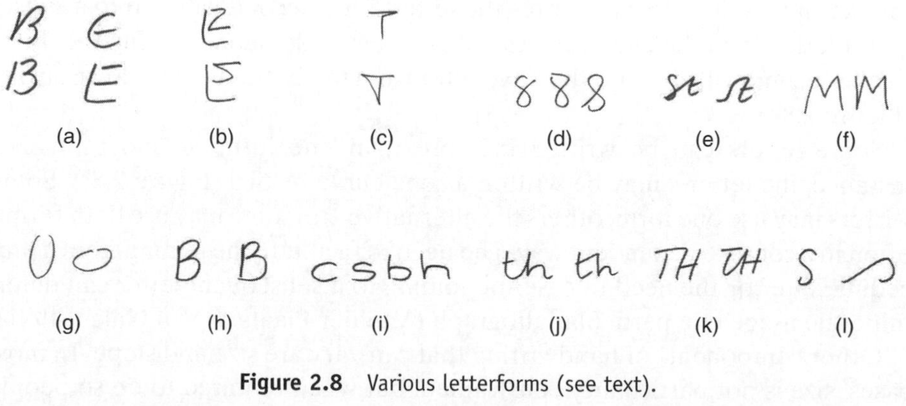

Figure 2.8 Various letterforms (see text).

fairly resistant to change. van Doorn and Keuss (1993), who focused on the repeated letter pair **lele**, found that there was a high level of spatial invariance when written under different circumstances (small, medium and large writing, with or without visual feedback).

Internal letter proportions are many and varied. For example, the letter **O** may be written as a tall, thin letter or as a squashed, flat letter (Figure 2.8g). This can be seen as a variation in proportion or as a variation in the shape of the letter. Another example of internal proportions would be the letter **B** with either both curved parts of roughly equal size or, as seen in many writers, the upper curve smaller than the lower curve (Figure 2.8h).

Some variations in proportion tend to occur in related groups of letters within the writing of the same person. For example, if a writer produces the letter **y** with a tail that is longer than the upper part of the letter, then it is likely that they will also produce the letters **g** and **p** in a similarly proportioned manner (Eldridge et al., 1985).

The shape of characters may also be connected; for example, a writer who produces a flattened, elongated form of the letter **c** may tend to produce a similarly flattened, elongated form of the letter **s**, and quite possibly the bowl elements of the letters **b** and **h** and so on (Figure 2.8i).

Thus, it can be seen that some features of writing tend to be somewhat generalised in the writing of a given person. This leads some to describe writing in very broad terms as, for example, rounded or angular.

Inter-character proportions vary too. The most common letter pair in English is **th**. In many writers, the two letters are of about equal height, but in a number of writers the **t** is routinely smaller than the **h** (Muehlberger et al., 1977). Not only can inter-letter proportions vary, so too can the way in which adjacent letters are joined. For instance, some writers join the letter **t** to the letter **h** via the tail of the **t**; others join to the letter **h** from the crossbar of the **t**, and some people do both (Figure 2.8j).

If capital letters are being hurriedly written, it is common for some letters to be joined. In this case, the joining often reflects the letter construction. So, for example, someone who writes the letter **T** top second will join to a subsequent letter from the end of the crossbar, whereas someone writing the down stroke second will join into the next letter from the bottom of the down stroke (Figure 2.8k).

Some letters can be written in more than one form or allograph. For instance, the letter **s** may be written as one curve or two (Figure 2.8l). Some writers may use one form, others the alternative and some may use both forms, often in a context-dependent way. The need to facilitate the joining from a preceding letter or the need to ease the joining to a subsequent letter can determine the usage of a particular allograph (Van der Plaats & Van Galen, 1991).

Other components of handwriting that can vary are size and slope. In most cases, size is not particularly constrained, but when required to do so people can make their writing either larger or smaller. When writing on a black-board, for example, the writing is not only larger but also requires the writer to adjust to writing on a different surface and at a different geometrical orientation to that usually used when writing at a desk. However, such changes do not significantly alter the appearance of the writing. Slope is fairly constant for some writers, but others may vary their slope markedly.

Another way of describing handwriting variation is to refer to schemes in which handwriting has been classified in some way. One such scheme was devised by Eldridge and colleagues (Eldridge et al., 1984) with the stated aim of focusing on the variability of handwriting both between and within writers. Its underlying purpose was to inform handwriting experts about feature frequency. The study considers the letters **d**, **f**, **h**, **k**, **p** and **t** and it examines these in requested samples from 61 adults, many of whom were from an educated background. The classification scheme used is very complex with often ten or more variants described for each letter. For example, the elements of the letter **f** are dissected by number of strokes (two categories), top of staff shape (three categories), top of staff direction (two categories), bottom of staff shape (three categories), bottom of staff direction (two categories), crossbar position (three categories) and crossbar curvature (three categories).

Similarly, Muehlberger et al. (1977) looked at the letter pair **th** because of its frequency of use in English. Their scheme also was complex and looked at the height ratio of the **th** (four categories), the shape of the **h** loop (five categories), shape of the **h** arch (three categories), height of the **t** crossbar (four categories), baseline of the **h** (four categories) and shape of the **t** (five categories). The purpose of such studies was to provide some statistical data on the features described and to point a way forward for similar research. However, such schemes can only describe a very limited amount of the variability to be found in handwriting, and for this reason they are not used routinely in casework.

Handwriting classification schemes have been devised for a variety of purposes. Some schemes use feature descriptors that are, as far as possible, mutually exclusive, typified by 'writer A uses form X' and 'writer B uses form Y' for a given letterform (for example, (Hardcastle et al., 1986). Whilst, *between-writer* variability is determined by such schemes, *within-writer* variability may not be quantified to give, for example, 'writer A uses form X 80% and form Y 20% of the time' and 'writer B uses the same two forms but form X 30% of the time and form Y 70% of the time'. In terms of writer identification, this more subtle view of variation is able to provide important additional information about the frequency of use of variants within the handwriting.

The diverse factors that affect the development of each person's handwriting from childhood to adulthood are, therefore, apparent in the basic letterforms used and the variations these show both between writers and within the handwriting from a single writer. The handwriting expert has to first observe these in samples of handwriting in casework and then has to interpret the significance of the observations in the context of each case situation. Studies of variation such as those mentioned above can help to provide some guide as to the frequency of occurrence of basic features in handwriting, but the subtleties of variability are much greater than such classification schemes can show, particularly when a single writer shows variation and different writers show different ranges of variation from one to another.

2.9   Interpretation of handwriting evidence

While close observation of the detail of handwriting is a necessary component of an effective forensic examination, it is not sufficient basis on its own to inevitably lead to a correct opinion of authorship being expressed. The link between observation and the resulting opinion is the interpretation phase of the examination. For a handwriting expert, interpretation requires experience to assess the significance of the many observations that are made, bringing together the various strands of the findings to reach a justifiable and defendable opinion that is capable of withstanding the glare of a court's spotlight as it seeks to assess the reliability of the handwriting expert's evidence.

Because interpretation is effectively a process that occurs in the expert's mind, it is difficult to devise procedures to ensure that the expert's thinking processes are correct. One way to gain confidence in an expert's view is for the interpretation process to be written down in the case notes, which can then be reviewed and checked independently by another expert. In other words, the checking procedure ensures that not only has a reasonable conclusion been expressed but also that the reasoning towards that conclusion is appropriate. If there is agreement in both of these elements then this provides reassurance and confidence that the first expert's interpretation is correct. Hence, the expert's opinion must contain elements that are capable of being demonstrated and explained so that there is a chain of evidence that can be followed and understood by others, from the question ('Who wrote the document in question?') to the opinion ('He did or did not'). It is not acceptable for experts to simply expect the courts to accept their opinion because it comes from an expert.

2.9.1   Limitations to the evidence in handwriting cases

If there are limitations to an examination, these must be indicated clearly and their impact on the interpretation reflected in the conclusion reached. There are many factors that can limit the effectiveness of a handwriting comparison. The most obvious are the amounts of questioned and specimen handwriting. Given the wide variety of handwriting features that are used, clearly the distinctiveness of the handwriting will play a part. If the handwriting is not very distinctive, incorporating many more frequently encountered letterforms, then it may be that it is possible to identify the author only after examining quite a lot of such handwriting and assessing the range of variation across many features present in the larger volume of writing. But if a piece of handwriting is more unusual then it may be possible to identify its author even from a relatively small amount.

If for a given writer certain letters and numerals are particularly distinctive, then their presence or absence in the case material may impact on the conclusion that can be reached. In other words, if the questioned handwriting consists of very distinctive numerals 4, 5 and 6, but the specimen only contains examples of 1, 2 and 3, then the fact that the questioned handwriting is distinctive is of little consequence in reaching a conclusion based on an unhelpful specimen.

The distinctiveness of handwriting is affected by the kinds of factor discussed in earlier sections of this chapter, especially where and when a person learned to write. Any tendency for certain handwriting features to be more (or less) common in particular groups of writers (from a particular country, for instance) obviously has the potential to affect the expert's view as to how unusual those features are. This all applies in particular to handwriting that has been naturally written. However, the writing process can be deliberately altered or disguised.

There are a number of commonly encountered strategies that are used when disguising handwriting. The nature and success of such strategies varies from person to person and so it is impossible to generalise on the effect the disguise will have. However, disguise is difficult to maintain due to the automaticity of handwriting in most adults. A deliberate, conscious effort to change handwriting may start off successfully, but as time passes there is almost always a tendency for the writer to revert back to their natural style. Of course, the writer may become aware of this and so it is common to see the level of disguise change over the document, sometimes more effective disguise, sometimes more natural. If it is possible to determine which are the more natural passages in the handwriting, for example those written with greater fluency or that are more 'normal' in appearance, then it may be possible for the expert to at least use these as more natural handwriting features.

The strategies used for disguise include some that are applied across all features, such as a change of slope or a change of size, some that are applied to related features, such as an exaggerated loop on letters such as **f**, **g** and **y**, and some that are letter specific, such as use of a completely different form of a letter. Use of the unaccustomed hand is sometimes attempted, but this is often apparent due to the lack of fluency this usually involves, since most writers are not able to write equally well with both hands. Skilful writers may attempt to disguise their handwriting by deliberately writing with less apparent skill and may also deliberately make the writing less literate by, for example, purposely misspelling words.

A change of writing implement can influence the appearance of handwriting, for example graffiti written with a paint brush on a wall as opposed to writing at a desk with a ballpoint pen on paper. Whether this is deliberate or simply a consequence of the case circumstances will depend on the situation.

Handwriting is affected by the age of the writer, particularly so in younger and older writers. In some cases this can limit the effectiveness of the comparison, especially if the questioned and specimen handwritings are not contemporary with one another. In those elderly people who have severe handwriting difficulty, the ability to write may change over very short periods of time and the variability of the handwriting may be so great that it is almost impossible to come to a firm conclusion no matter how much specimen handwriting is obtained.

Observations of the handwriting and interpretation of their significance in the light of any limitations lead to a conclusion that must take account of alternative explanations for the observations. This approach to interpretation will now be discussed.

2.9.2   Reaching conclusions

Over the years a number of ways of looking at the interpretation of forensic evidence has been advocated. A detailed discussion of this topic can be found, for example, in Aitken and Taroni (2004). However, the handwriting expert generally has to consider a small number of possible situations with regard to the examination – often simply coming down to (i) the suspect did write the document in question or (ii) the suspect did not write the document in question. The expert must weigh the findings (derived from the observations) against the competing propositions with a view to determining which is best supported by the findings. It is not necessarily the case that all the findings will point in the same direction. Rather, it is sometimes the case that at least some findings will support one proposition and others an alternative proposition. In addition, some findings will be more significant than others and thus carry more weight when deciding which of the competing propositions is best supported by the overall evidence. Knowledge of how handwriting is likely to vary, the effects of age and the effects of where and when people were taught to write – all of the factors discussed in this chapter – inform the handwriting expert's interpretation in each casework situation.

The limitations of the case often affect the degree of certainty with which the expert is able to reach a conclusion. Forensic evidence is not required to be black or white. Indeed the courts require expert witnesses to be able to express an opinion and this often involves a view on how likely alternative explanations are. This must all be conveyed carefully in the wording of the report and for this reason it is common practice to have a scale of opinions that reflects the degrees of certainty available.

There have been various scales put forward over the years but most capture at least four levels of opinion and some have several more. The four major points on the scale consist of:

- **Conclusive** opinions, where the evidence is so overwhelming that only one interpretation is acceptable, with the alternative(s) being so unlikely that they can be discounted.

- Sometimes the evidence falls a little short of this very high standard, often as a result of case limitations, and in this circumstance the evidence is typically described as **strong** with alternative(s) being **unlikely** but not so unlikely as to be discounted – in other words there is a small element of doubt.

- If the evidence is weaker still but with one explanation being somewhat more likely than other explanation(s), but the other explanations not being by any means capable of being ruled out, then the evidence is often described as **weak** – in other words it is indicating which evidence, **on balance**, is the most likely given the observations and limitations.

- Finally, in some cases the evidence is too close to call for the expert to come to a conclusion at all, in which case the evidence is **inconclusive** and no alternative is favoured above any other and so the evidence could be regarded as neutral.

Opinions that fall short of conclusive are not an admission of failure by the expert to 'get the right answer' but rather are a very important part of the expert's role in determining the strength of evidence available from the material examined. Because of the nature of the interpretation process by the expert, it is perhaps not surprising that the use of computers to assist in the decision-making process in handwriting comparisons has been advocated, and this will be looked at next.

2.9.3 Computer use in interpretation

In the field of automated handwriting recognition, much work has been done to try to describe the written line as a mathematical function. In order to analyse handwriting mathematically, there are two components that can be measured. The first is the static component, which is the image of the completed handwriting or signature. The second component is the dynamic component, which can measure parameters such as the dimensions of the signature, the length of the written line, pen velocity over the paper, times when the pen is lifted from the paper and the pen pressure. Further measures can be calculated from these, such as the acceleration of the pen as it speeds up after starting a pen stroke and slows down as it comes towards the end of the pen stroke. Devices capable of measuring the dynamic components of handwriting and signature production are usually known as handwriting tablets (see Box 2.2).

Bridging the divide between this work and the classification of writing are studies such as that of Marquis et al. (2005), which uses mathematical techniques to convert shapes of handwriting on the page into mathematical expressions. Using this kind of approach, they showed that the letters **O** from three writers were different in their mathematical form. There was variation within the mathematical renditions and thus the possibility of 'misattributing' outliers, when looking at single examples, cannot be ruled out. Further work by Marquis and colleagues looked at similarly analysed transformations of the loops of the letters **a**, **d**, **o** and **q** from 13 writers (Marquis et al., 2006). They found discrimination values of about 70–80% for the letters **a**, **d**, **o** and **q**. Different loops were found to have different values for discriminating between different pairs of writers, as would be expected from the complex nature of writing. For example, the shape of the loop of the letter **o** was less discriminating than the loop shape of the other three letters studied, whereas the shape of the loop of the letter **d** was the best at discriminating between writers.

In a similar vein, Ling (Ling, 2002) measured 10 elements of cursive writing, such as word spacing, the space between the ascenders of the letters **t** and **h** in the **th** letter pair, the space between the sides of the letter **u** and so on. Ling also found that no one feature was able to provide discrimination between the writings of the 10 participants. Rather, he finds that a feature that discriminates between two given writers may not be so useful when discriminating between two other writers or even one of the original pair and a third writer.

A number of studies, such as that of Srihari and colleagues (Srihari et al., 2002), has shown that various algorithms can be used to examine handwriting samples offline (that is, from the static image rather than the additional dynamic information that can be obtained using a digitising tablet). The purpose of his study was to test the hypothesis of handwriting individuality in adult handwriting, a hypothesis that has come under scrutiny following various legal challenges to expert evidence in handwriting in the USA, summarised in Srihari et al. (2002). As Srihari recognises, the algorithms used may share some elements with those that forensic experts use, but they are not identical with them.

How do studies that aim to convert handwriting into mathematical constructs link in with classification studies that have the same aim, namely to give more objective data of the frequency of occurrence of handwriting features? Even the simple **th** letter join studied by Muehlberger and colleagues

(Muehlberger et al., 1977) produced a detailed series of categories that over-lapped depending on the variants present in a person's handwriting. Looked at in another way, given the advances in computing power in the years since such observation-based schemes were proposed, the absence of a computer-based approach to solving forensic handwriting problems is notable.

It is worth mentioning parallel studies that have attracted a lot of interest and that are aimed at handwriting recognition in the sense of determining what has been written, so that handwriting can be converted automatically to computer text, for example on hand-held devices with a stylus input. That there is a need for such conversion is interesting as it implies that there is still an advantage to handwriting in many circumstances, albeit clearly less need for it with the dominance of the computer keyboard, and indeed computers that have increasing capabilities of voice recognition. Contemporary studies of the amount of handwriting done by people of different ages shows that there is still a value in being able to write (van Drempt et al., 2011).

Such computer-centred studies have added support for the individualisa-tion hypothesis. However, forensic casework is constrained by the real world and does not operate in the experimental laboratory. This is a crucial limita-tion on the applicability of the results of such studies. In essence, going from the general to the particular is fraught with danger. And computers are not (yet) able to factor in such human dimensions as intended disguise, the effects of intoxicants or the effects of illness on handwriting.

The value of computer-based studies is that they can help to contribute to the conclusions reached by handwriting experts about individuality, but it would be unwise to let computers replace the handwriting expert until such time that it can be shown that they can outperform the human expert across the range of case types encountered (Srihari & Singer, 2014).

2.10 Examination notes in handwriting cases

When examining any case forensically it is important to make full and comprehensive notes about what has been observed, what significance has been attached to the observations, what possible explanations have been considered and the conclusions reached. This provides an audit trail from the question to the conclusion and its description in the notes should be a close reflection of the observations and thoughts of the expert, providing evidence that the opinion has been reached in a logical and robust way.

There are many ways of making case notes in handwriting cases. Many handwriting experts will sketch out the handwriting features in order to clearly show their form, which may not be obvious and may require magnification and interpretation of pen movement. Further, the act of sketching emphasises the structure and proportions of all of the elements of the text and may also give an indication of how easy or complex the execution of the handwriting is and hence how distinctive it is. An alternative is to photocopy the handwriting of interest and to annotate it in such a way as to again make the features and their structure clear. The purpose of these notes is to dissect the formation of the handwriting and to record it to make it plain what has been seen by the expert during the examination.

If the amount of handwriting is fairly small then it may be best to sketch or note all of the handwriting, but as the amount of handwriting increases this becomes impractical, due to constraints of time, and pointless when it is clear that the handwriting is by a single writer. Instead, the expert may create a body of handwriting, or group of handwriting, that shows consistent and significant connections within itself so as to be considered as having been written by just one person. Of course, any deviations from the group must be noted as they may well indicate one or more other writers being involved. Making notes about a group of handwriting inevitably requires the expert to note the formation of a selection of examples from the larger body of handwriting present. The selected features noted must be representative of the formation of the feature in the whole body of handwriting. Typically this might mean noting several key variants of a letter to show how the writer forms it in most instances, together with any significant departures from this pattern where the writer for some reason uses a less frequently used variation. When complete, the notes contain a record of the variability of all of the handwriting features present. This is a snapshot of the total output of handwriting from a given writer, but given the habitual nature of handwriting this can be taken into account by an expert familiar with how people's handwriting varies in different circumstances.

A comparison is made between the handwriting in question and a specimen of handwriting, feature by feature and noting any similarities or differences. If the amount of questioned handwriting is small then each and every letter and number present can be compared. But if there is a lot of handwriting in question, then the group formed to reflect the variations present can be compared with the specimen, albeit it remains possible to compare specific parts of the questioned handwriting with the specimen if needed.

Comparison of handwriting features can be recorded in a number of ways. Given the inherent variability of handwriting, it is not appropriate to look for absolutely identical (superimposable) levels of similarity. Rather, a scale of perhaps four levels of similarity can be used. A very close match would form the greatest degree of similarity; a reasonably close match would form the next level and would indicate a fairly small and probably minor difference; the next level would be a fairly major difference and could be indicative of having another writer; and a major, significant difference would strongly suggest a second writer.

The significance of these levels of similarity and difference between a piece of questioned handwriting and a specimen will be determined by an *overall* assessment of them *collectively*, a process that draws heavily on the experience of the expert. The expert will need to weigh up the evidence provided by the observations of the handwriting in light of the many factors that were discussed earlier in the chapter. In that context, the expert should decide which similarities and differences are the more important and which therefore are key to the conclusion being reached.

Making good examination notes is not, however, a guarantee that the expert will come to the correct conclusion, though it is made more likely since the observations and thought processes are recorded and articulated. The final interpretation stage is where authorship is attributed (or not) to a given writer. The process is helped by experts using the scale of opinion described in Section 2.9.2. By the very nature of the range of handwriting examinations, it is impossible to give standard conditions that form the basis of these levels of opinion. The observations and their interpretation all need to be noted, showing clearly which elements are the most important to the decision reached and in the context of relevant limitations, hence justifying the opinion level used.

2.11 Reporting findings

The purpose of the examination, even if it seems very obvious, should nonetheless be stated unambiguously. This sets out the context for what will follow in terms of findings and conclusions.

The findings should be described stating what has been found as a result of the examination. The amount of detail given in reports varies between experts but it should at least indicate what the findings are, such as whether there are significant similarities (or differences) between the questioned and specimen handwritings. Any limitations to the examination should also be described since these will probably lead to the justification of a qualified opinion being expressed.

The conclusion is given finally and includes an assessment of how likely other explanations for the findings are given the findings and the limitations in the case. It is also good practice to end the report with a short summary that states the key conclusions so the reader can quickly see them and can refer to the body of the report for their reasons.

These are the main requirements of written reports but there may be additional requirements for reports or statements written in various judicial circumstances, which vary between different countries.

Often the main focus of attention in cases involving handwriting is the signature rather than any other handwriting, since the signature has special significance and because of this is much more likely to be simulated by another person attempting to copy it and pass it off as genuine. The examination of signatures will be considered in Chapter 3.

Handwriting comparison: a worked example

In this section an example of how to approach a case and make notes is demonstrated. The worked example is intended to show a general process in terms of thinking and doing, rather than an expectation that the reader will 'test' themselves to see if they can get the 'right' answer (although getting the 'right' answer could be regarded as a welcome bonus!).

It should be stressed that there are a number of different ways to make notes but the intention here is to show the kinds of issues that need to be considered and how these inter-relate with the observation process leading to a conclusion.

Case circumstances

An anonymous note has been recovered from the scene of a burglary. Items taken from the burglary were subsequently recovered from the home of the suspect. A small handwriting sample has been obtained at request from the suspect who then refused to provide any more handwriting.

Purpose

To compare the questioned handwriting on the anonymous note with the handwriting sample from the suspect to determine the authorship of the note.

Items submitted

Item 1: Anonymous note (Figure 2.9)

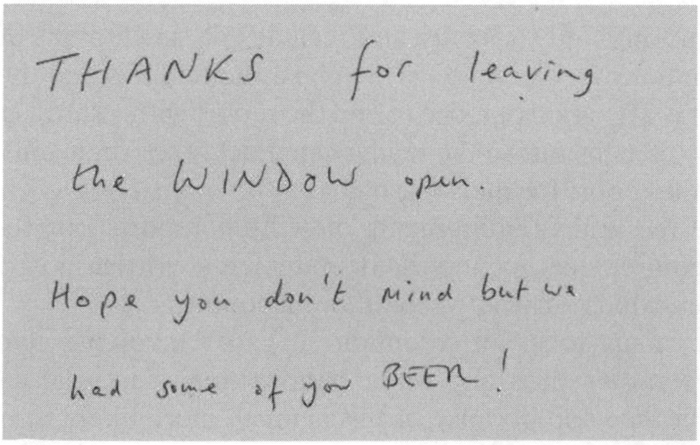

Figure 2.9   Worked example: Anonymous note.

Item 2: Sample of handwriting (Figure 2.10)

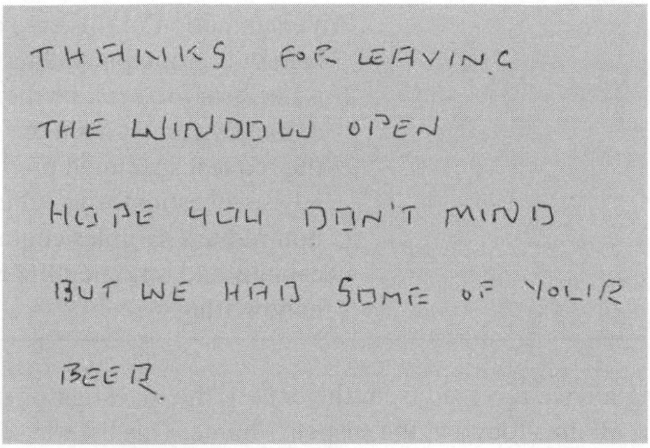

THANKS FOR LEAVING

THE WINDOW OPEN

HOPE YOU DON'T MIND

BUT WE HAD SOME OF YOUR

BEER.

Figure 2.10 Worked example: Sample of handwriting.

Case notes

Observations	Thoughts
Examination of the questioned handwriting shows mix of some capitals and some unjoined lower case writing.	Handwriting perhaps looks contrived (so not completely natural?) but with one or two natural features such as t-h join and the E-R join.
Fluency appears to be reasonable – evidence is tailing off of pen line, such as end of R in BEER, flick at end of second W of WINDOW and general variable pen pressure showing pen moving quickly.	Not much handwriting in question so will be difficult to form a strong conclusion. But fluent so may be able to provide some supporting evidence (positive or negative)?
The specimen handwriting looks very unnatural, evidence such as use of 'squared' letters **O**, **A** and **D**. No lower case writing in sample.	This specimen is inadequate because (i) it is not natural, (ii) even if it was naturally written it does not contain enough handwriting to show natural variation, (iii) it does not contain lower case handwriting.

Observations	Thoughts
	An examination of this case as it stands cannot in principle yield a result.
	It is necessary to seek further samples of handwriting. Given the nature of the request specimen provided here, advise investigator to submit any non-request samples containing capitals and unjoined lower case handwriting.

Following advice received from the expert, the investigator submitted a list of music albums found at the suspect's home. This list was identified by the suspect's former girlfriend as having been written by the suspect. The suspect made no comment when asked about the authorship of the list.

Further item submitted

Item 3: List of music albums (Figure 2.11)

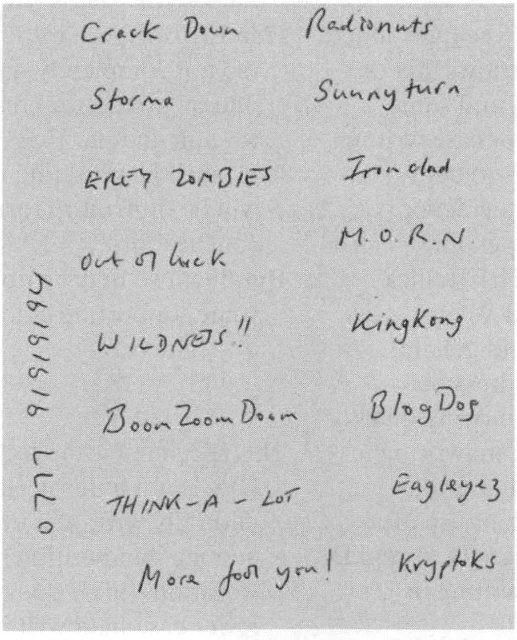

Figure 2.11 Worked example: List of music albums.

Observations	Thoughts
Music list contains mix of capitals and unjoined lower case letters. Appears natural.	This is more helpful as a specimen as it appears more natural and is fluently written. But is it all written by one person? What about numerals in margin? Look for features that link or do not link the entries.
Initial examination shows many cross-linking features such as K (in THINK, KingKong and Kryptoks; B in ZOMBIES and Boom; R in Radionuts and M.O.R.N; t in Stoma and Kryproks.	Preliminary evidence points to list having been written by one person with no obvious exception. No numerals within list to compare with entry in margin. No numerals in questioned document anyway so safe to exclude numerals in margin as unexamined as they are irrelevant. Most letters in questioned note are present in the specimen handwriting. Can now make full examination of questioned and specimen handwriting and make comparison.
Make detailed notes, including sketches, of *questioned* handwriting showing structure. Note: • pen type and ink colour • fluency • structure of individual letters and how they join • distinctiveness and amount of handwriting.	Ink is blue ballpoint ink (microscopy shows oily ink deposit with striations). Fluency appears to be reasonable – evidence is tailing off of pen line such as end of R in BEER, flick at end of second W of WINDOW and general variable pen pressure showing pen moving quickly. Fairly small amount of handwriting in question. Features such as K, S, D, B, E-R join, t-h join, f, y, and a are notable. No one feature is unique but in combination it is fairly distinctive handwriting.

Observations	Thoughts
Make detailed notes, including sketches, of *specimen* handwriting showing structure. Note: • pen type and ink colour • fluency • structure of individual letters and how they join • distinctiveness and amount of handwriting.	Ink is black ballpoint ink (microscopy shows oily ink deposit with striations). All entries similar colour – no need to examine further at this stage. Fluency appears to be reasonable – similar kinds of evidence as for the questioned handwriting. More specimen than questioned handwriting. Full comparison to see if all by one person and to compare with questioned handwriting.

Having carefully determined the structure of the questioned and specimen handwritings separately, the next stage is to compare them. Some features may correspond closely, others may not. The significance of features is interpreted based on the expert's experience. In the following, features are not identified as being significant or not but the key point is that these assessments must be documented.

Observations	Thoughts
Annotate sketches of questioned handwriting showing whether the features are similar to or different from those in the specimen handwriting. This should show the following: • There are some significant similarities between the questioned handwriting on item 1 and the specimen of handwriting item 3. They include the following letters: ***. • There are some features of the questioned handwriting that are not so well matched in the specimen. They include ***. • The following features are present on the questioned item but are absent from the specimen: ***.	What are the possible explanations? 1. The questioned note was written by the suspect. 2. The questioned note was *not* written by the suspect. 3. The questioned note was written by someone trying to copy the suspect's handwriting (a theoretical possibility but since it was written seemingly at the scene of a burglary and the handwriting on item 1 seems fluent, this possibility is very remote and would be extremely unusual).

Observations	Thoughts
(In the expert's opinion) the similarities are significant and the differences are minor. Taking this into account together with the amounts of handwriting and its overall distinctiveness the conclusion is …	Alternative 1 is supported by the significant similarities found. Alternative 2 is less likely than alternative 1 because such a degree of similarity occurring by chance with some other person's handwriting would be a very considerable coincidence which is unlikely to happen. Alternative 3 is also unlikely given the case situation and the fluency of the handwriting in question.
	Alternative 1 is the best explanation for the findings and the other alternatives are much less likely.
	What strength of evidence is justified in this case?
	A conclusive opinion is not safe given the few unmatched features, lack of distinctiveness and small amounts of handwriting. To discount another writer on the evidence available could not be justified.
	A strong opinion is justified by the significant similarities and absence of major differences. It is unlikely that some other by chance has such a similar style of handwriting.
	A limited opinion would be understating the available evidence.
Summary	There is strong but not conclusive evidence that the questioned handwriting on item 1 was written by the same person that wrote the list, item 3, and it is unlikely that some other person did so. The key features are ***.

Report of Forensic Expert

(Again, it is stressed that this report is intended to demonstrate an approach and not to be a test of getting the 'right' answer.)

Qualifications and experience ...

Scope of expertise ...

Items examined

I have examined the following items at the instruction of (the investigating authority). They were received at the laboratory on (dates).

Item 1: Questioned note

Item 2: Specimen of handwriting

Item 3: List of music

Purpose

I have compared the questioned handwriting on item 1 with the specimens of handwriting, items 2 and 3, with a view to determining the authorship of item 1.

Findings

The specimen of handwriting, item 2, is unnatural in appearance and I have not used it in my examination.

The list of music, item 3, shows similar handwriting throughout and I can accept that has been written by one and the same person. I have taken this to be a specimen attributable to X (suspect).

I note that the numerals in the left margin of item 3 cannot be compared to the other details on item 3 and there are no numerals in question on item 1, I have therefore not used these numerals in my examination.

There are some significant similarities between the questioned handwriting and the specimen of handwriting in the list of music on item 3. However, there are also a few features that are not well matched and the questioned handwriting is limited in amount and not especially distinctive. For these reasons a conclusive opinion of authorship cannot be expressed, but the similarities found, in my opinion, provide strong evidence that X wrote the note in question and it is unlikely that some other person did so.

Summary

There are some significant similarities between the questioned handwriting on the note and the list of music on item 3 which, in my opinion, provide strong evidence that they were written by one and the same person.

References

Aitken, C., & Taroni, F. (2004). *Statistics and the Evaluation of Evidence for Forensic Scientists* (Second edition). London: John Wiley and Sons Ltd.

Allen, M. (2011). *Developmental Aspects of Handwriting Acquisition*. Staffordshire University.

Arter, C., McCall, S., & Bowyer, T. (1996). Handwriting and children with visual impairments. *British Journal of Special Education*, 23(1), 25–28. doi:10.1111/j.1467-8578.1996.tb00939.x.

Asicioglu, F., & Turan, N. (2003). Handwriting changes under the effect of alcohol. *Forensic Science International*, 132(3), 201–210. doi:10.1016/S0379-0738(03)00020-3 ER

Baddeley, A. (2003). Working memory: Looking back and looking forward. *Nature Reviews Neuroscience*, 4(10), 829–839. doi:10.1038/nrn1201.

Balestrino, M., Fontana, P., Terzuoli, S., et al. (2012). Altered handwriting suggests cognitive impairment and may be relevant to posthumous evaluation. *Journal of Forensic Sciences*, 57(5), 1252–1258. doi:10.1111/j.1556-4029.2012.02131.x.

Beck, J. (1985). Handwriting of the alcoholic. *Forensic Science International*, 28(1), 19–26. doi:10.1016/0379-0738(85)90161-6.

Berninger, V. W., Abbott, R. D., Swanson, H. L., et al. (2010). Relationship of word- and sentence-level working memory to reading and writing in second, fourth, and sixth grade. *Language Speech and Hearing Services in Schools*, 41(2), 179–193. doi:10.1044/0161-1461(2009/08-0002).

Blote, A. W., & Hamstra-Bletz, L. (1991). A longitudinal study on the structure of handwriting. *Perceptual Motor Skills*, 72(8), 983–994.

Bonoti, F., Vlachos, F., & Metallidou, P. (2005). Writing and drawing performance of school age children : Is there any relationship? *School Psychology International*, 26(2), 243–255. doi:10.1177/0143034305052916.

Bryant, M. S., Rintala, D. H., Lai, E. C., & Protas, E. J. (2010). An investigation of two interventions for micrographia in individuals with Parkinson's disease. *Clinical Rehabilitation*, 24(11), 1021–1026. doi:10.1177/0269215510371420.

Bumin, G., & Kavak, S. T. (2010). An investigation of the factors affecting handwriting skill in children with hemiplegic cerebral palsy (vol 30, pg 1374, 2008). *Disability and Rehabilitation*, 32(8), 692–703. doi:10.3109/09638281003654789.

Burger, D. K., & McCluskey, A. (2011). Australian norms for handwriting speed in healthy adults aged 60-99 years. *Australian Occupational Therapy Journal*, 58(5), 355–363. doi:10.1111/j.1440-1630.2011.00955.x.

Burton, A. W., & Dancisak, M. J. (2000). Grip form and graphomotor control in preschool children. *American Journal of Occupational Therapy*, 54(1), 9–17. doi:10.5014/ajot.54.1.9.

Cheng, N., Gek, K. L., Bei, S. Y., et al. (2005). Investigation of class characteristics in English handwriting of the three main racial groups: Chinese, Malay and Indian in Singapore. *Journal of Forensic Sciences*, 50(1), 177–184.

Chiappedi, M., Togni, R., De Bernardi, E., et al. (2012). Arm trajectories and writing strategy in healthy children. *BMC Pediatrics*, 12, 173. doi:10.1186/1471-2431-12-173.

Croisile, B. (1999). Agraphia in Alzheimer's disease. *Dementia and Geriatric Cognitive Disorders*, 10(3), 226–230. doi:10.1159/000017124.

Cusack, C. T., & Hargett, J. W. (1989). A comparison study of the handwriting of adolescents. *Forensic Science International*, 42(3), 239–248. doi:10.1016/0379-0738(89)90091-1.

Debastiani, P., & Barry, C. (1989). A cognitive analysis of an acquired dysgraphic patient with an allographic writing disorder. *Cognitive Neuropsychology*, 6(1), 25–41. doi:10.1080/02643298908253283.

Destreri, N. D., Farina, E., Alberoni, M., et al. (2000). Selective uppercase dysgraphia with loss of visual imagery of letter forms: A window on the organization of graphomotor patterns. *Brain and Language*, 71(3), 353–372.

Dhawn, B. N., Bapat, S. K., & Saxena, V. C. (1969). Effect of four centrally acting drugs on handwriting. *Japanese Journal of Pharmacology*, 19(1), 63–7. doi:10.1254/jjp.19.63.

Eldridge, M. A., Nimmo-Smith, I., Wing, A. M., & Totty, R. N. (1984). The variability of selected features in cursive handwriting: Categorical measures. *Journal of the Forensic Science Society*, 24(3), 179–219.

Eldridge, M. A., Nimmo-Smith, I., Wing, A. M., & Totty, R. N. (1985). The dependence between selected categorical measures of cursive handwriting. *Journal of the Forensic Science Society*, 25(3), 217–231.

Ellen, D. (2006). *Scientific Examination of Documents Methods and Techniques* (3rd edition). London: CRC Press.

Ericsson, K., Forssell, L. G., Holmen, K., et al. (1996). Copying and handwriting ability in the screening of cognitive dysfunction in old age. *Archives of Gerontology and Geriatrics*, 22(2), 103–121. doi:10.1016/0167-4943(95)00685-0.

Feder, K. P., & Majnemer, A. (2007). Handwriting development, competency, and intervention. *Developmental Medicine and Child Neurology*, 49(4), 312–317.

Fodor, J. A. (1983). *Modularity of Mind*. London: MIT Press.

Fuentes, C. T., Mostofsky, S. H., & Bastian, A. J. (2010). Perceptual reasoning predicts handwriting impairments in adolescents with autism. *Neurology*, 75(20), 1825–1829. doi:10.1212/WNL.0b013e3181fd633d.

Galbraith, N. G. (1986). Alcohol - its effect on handwriting. *Journal of Forensic Sciences*, 31(2), 580–588.

Graham, S., Struck, M., Santoro, J., & Berninger, V. W. (2006). Dimensions of good and poor handwriting legibility in first and second graders: Motor programs, visual-spatial arrangement, and letter formation parameter setting. *Developmental Neuropsychology*, 29(1), 43–60.

Graham, S., Weintraub, N., & Berninger, V. W. (1998). The relationship between handwriting style and speed and legibility. *Journal of Educational Research*, 91(5), 290–296.

Graham, S., Weintraub, N., Schafer, W., & Berninger, V. (1998). Development of handwriting speed and legibility in grades 1-9. *Journal of Educational Research*, 92(1), 42–52.

Gregg, L.W. and Steinberg, E. R. (1980). *Cognitive Processes in Writing* (1st edition). New Jersey: Lawrence Erlbaum Associates.

Hammerschmidt, S. L., & Sudsawad, P. (2004). Teachers' survey on problems with handwriting: Referral, evaluation, and outcomes. *American Journal of Occupational Therapy*, 58(2), 185–192.

Hardcastle, R. A., Thornton, D., & Totty, R. N. (1986). A computer-based system for the classification of handwriting on cheques. *Journal of the Forensic Science Society*, 26(3), 383–392.

Hollis, S., & Low, J. (2005). Karmiloff-Smith's RRM distinction between adjunctions and redescriptions: It's about time (and children's drawings). *British Journal of Developmental Psychology*, 23(4), 623–644.

Hoy, M. M. P., Egan, M. Y., & Feder, K. P. (2011). A systematic review of interventions to improve handwriting. *Canadian Journal of Occupational Therapy-Revue Canadienne D Ergotherapie*, 78(1), 13–25. doi:10.2182/cjot.2011.78.1.3.

Huber, R. A., & Headrick, A. M. (Eds). (1999). *Handwriting Identification: Facts and Fundamentals* (1st edition). New York: CRC Press.

Kaiser, M., Albaret, J., & Doudin, P. (2009). Relationship between visual-motor integration, eye-hand coordination, and quality of handwriting. *Journal of Occupational Therapy, Schools, & Early Intervention*, 2(2), 95. Retrieved from http://www.informaworld.com/10.1080/19411240903146228

Kandel, S., Álvarez, C. J., & Vallée, N. (2006). Syllables as processing units in handwriting production. *Journal of Experimental Psychology: Human Perception and Performance*, 32(1), 18–31. doi:10.1037/0096-1523.32.1.18.

Kellogg, R. (1969). *Analyzing Children's Art*. Mountain View, California: Mayfield Publishing Company.

Koziatek, S. M., & Powell, N. (2002). A validity study of the evaluation tool of children's handwriting - cursive. *American Journal of Occupational Therapy*, 56(4), 446–453.

Ling, S. (2002). A preliminary investigation into handwriting examination by multiple measurements of letters and spacing. *Forensic Science International*, 126(2), 145–149. doi:DOI: 10.1016/S0379-0738(02)00048-8.

Longstaff, M. G., & Heath, R. A. (2003). The influence of motor system degradation on the control of handwriting movements: A dynamical systems analysis. *Human Movement Science*, 22(1), 91–110.

Margolin, D. I., & Wing, A. M. (1983). Agraphia and micrographia - clinical manifestations of motor programming and performance disorders. *Acta Psychologica*, 54(1–3), 263–283. doi:10.1016/0001-6918(83)90039-2.

Marquis, R., Schmittbuhl, M., Mazzella, W. D., & Taroni, F. (2005). Quantification of the shape of handwritten characters: A step to objective discrimination between writers based on the study of the capital character O. *Forensic Science International*, 150(1), 23–32. doi:10.1016/j.forsciint.2004.06.028.

Marquis, R., Taroni, F., Bozza, S., & Schmittbuhl, M. (2006). Quantitative characterization of morphological polymorphism of handwritten characters loops. *Forensic Science International*, 164(2–3), 211–220. doi: 10.1016/j.forsciint.2006.02.008.

Marr, D., Windsor, M., & Cermak, S. (2001). Handwriting readiness: Locatives and visuomotor skills in the kindergarten year. *Early Childhood Research and Practice*, 34, 1–28.

Masson, J. F. (1988). Deciphering the handwriting of the recently blinded - a case-study. *Forensic Science International*, 38(3–4), 161–171. doi:10.1016/0379-0738(88)90163-6.

Mathyer, J. (1969). The influence of writing instruments on handwriting and signatures. *The Journal of Criminal Law, Criminology, and Police Science*, 60(1), 102–112. Retrieved from http://www.jstor.org/stable/1141743

Mavrogiorgou, P., Mergl, R., Tigges, P., et al. (2001). Kinematic analysis of handwriting movements in patients with obsessive-compulsive disorder. *Journal of Neurology Neurosurgery and Psychiatry*, 70(5), 605–612. doi:10.1136/jnnp.70.5.605.

McCutchen, D. (2000). Knowledge, processing, and working memory: Implications for a theory of writing. *Educational Psychologist*, 35(1), 13–23.

Mechtcheriakov, S., Graziadei, I. W., Kugener, A., et al. (2006). Motor dysfunction in patients with liver cirrhosis: Impairment of handwriting. *Journal of Neurology*, 253(3), 349–356. doi:10.1007/s00415-005-0995-5.

Meulenbroek, R. G. J., & Van Galen, G. P. (1989). Variations in cursive handwriting performance as a function of handedness, hand posture and gender. *Journal of Human Movement Studies*, 16(5), 239–254.

Miller, P. H. (2002). Order in variability, variability in order - why it matters for theories of development. *Human Development*, 45(3), 161–166.

Morasso, P., Ivaldi, F. A. M., & Ruggiero, C. (1983). How a discontinuous mechanism can produce continuous patterns in trajectory formation and handwriting. *Acta Psychologica*, 54(1–3), 83–98.

Muehlberger, R. J., Newman, K. W., Regent, J., & Wichmann, J. G. (1977). A statistical examination of selected handwriting characteristics. *Journal of Forensic Sciences*, 22(1), 206–215.

Naider-Steinhart, S., & Katz-Leurer, M. (2007). Analysis of proximal and distal muscle activity during handwriting tasks. *American Journal of Occupational Therapy*, 61(4), 392–398.

Perrin, M., Cordato, D. J., Fung, V. S., & Wong, D. (2005). Acute and reversible micrographia in a patient possibly due to cerebral ischaemia. *Journal of Clinical Neuroscience*, 12(3), 329–331. doi:10.1016/j.jocn.2004.05.004.

Phelps, J., Stempel, L., & Speck, G. (1985). The children's handwriting scale - a new diagnostic-tool. *Journal of Educational Research*, 79(1), 46–50.

Phillips, J. G., Ogeil, R. P., & Mueller, F. (2009). Alcohol consumption and handwriting: A kinematic analysis. *Human Movement Science*, 28(5), 619–632. doi:10.1016/j.humov .2009.01.006.

Poluha, P. C., Teulings, H. L., & Brookshire, R. H. (1998). Handwriting and speech changes across the levodopa cycle in Parkinson's disease. *Acta Psychologica*, 100(1–2), 71–84. doi:10.1016/S0001-6918(98)00026-2.

Richards, T. L., Berninger, V. W., Stock, P., et al. (2011). Differences between good and poor child writers on fMRI contrasts for writing newly taught and highly practiced letter forms. *Reading and Writing*, 24(5), 493–516. doi:10.1007/s11145-009-9217-3.

Rosenblum, S., & Weiss, P. L. (2010). Evaluating functional decline in patients with multiple sclerosis. *Research in Developmental Disabilities*, 31(2), 577–586. doi:10.1016/j.ridd .2009.12.008.

Rueckriegel, S. M., Blankenburg, F., Burghardt, R., et al. (2008). Influence of age and movement complexity on kinematic hand movement parameters in childhood and adolescence. *International Journal of Developmental Neuroscience*, 26(7), 655–663.

Sassoon, R. (1990). *Handwriting: The Way to Teach It*. Cheltenham: Stanley Thomas.

Schneck, C. M., & Henderson, A. (1990). Descriptive analysis of the developmental progression of grip position for pencil and crayon control in nondysfunctional children. *The American Journal of Occupational Therapy*, 44(10), 893–900.

Siebner, H. R., Limmer, C., Peinemann, A., et al. (2002). Long-term consequences of switching handedness: A positron emission tomography study on handwriting in 'converted' left-handers. *The Journal of Neuroscience*, 22(7), 2816–2825.

Siegler, R. S. (2002). Variability and infant development. *Infant Behavior & Development*, 25(4), 550–557.

Srihari, S. N., Cha, S. H., Arora, H., & Lee, S. (2002). Individuality of handwriting. *Journal of Forensic Sciences*, 47(4), 856–872.

Srihari, S. N., & Singer, K. (2014). Role of automation in the examination of handwritten items. *Pattern Recognition*, 47(3), 1083–1095. doi:10.1016/j.patcog.2013.09.032.

Summers, J. (2001). Joint laxity in the index finger and thumb and its relationship to pencil grasps used by children. *Australian Occupational Therapy Journal*, 48(3), 132–141.

Thomassen, A. J. W. M., Meulenbroek, R. G. J., & Tibosch, H. J. C. M. (1991). Latencies and kinematics reflect graphic production rules. *Human Movement Science*, 10(2–3), 271–289.

Tseng, M. H. (1998). Development of pencil grip position in preschool children. *The Occupational Therapy Journal of Research*, 18(4), 207–224.

Tucha, O., & Lange, K. W. (2004). Effects of nicotine chewing gum on a real-life motor task: A kinematic analysis of handwriting movements in smokers and non-smokers. *Psychopharmacology*, 173(1–2), 49–56. doi:10.1007/s00213-003-1690-9.

Tucha, O., Mecklinger, L., Thome, J., et al. (2006a). Kinematic analysis of dopaminergic effects on skilled handwriting movements in Parkinson's disease. *Journal of Neural Transmission*, 113(5), 609–623. doi:10.1007/s00702-005-0346-9.

Tucha, O., Walitza, S., Mecklinger, L., et al. (2006b). The effect of caffeine on handwriting movements in skilled writers. *Human Movement Science*, 25(4–5), 523–535. doi:10.1016/j.humov.2006.06.001.

Turnbull, S. J., Jones, A. E., & Allen, M. (2010). Identification of the class characteristics in the handwriting of polish people writing in English. *Journal of Forensic Sciences*, 55(5), 1296–1303. doi:10.1111/j.1556-4029.2010.01449.x ER.

Ueda, K., Matsuo, K., & Schwid, B. L. (2009). Experimental analysis of individuality of Japanese handwriting. *International Journal of Pattern Recognition and Artificial Intelligence*, 23(5), 869–885. doi:10.1142/S0218001409007545.

Van der Plaats, R. E., & Van Galen, G. P. (1991). Allographic variability in adult handwriting. *Human Movement Science*, 10(2–3), 291–300.

van Doorn, R. R. A., & Keuss, P. J. G. (1993). Spatial invariance of handwriting. *Reading and Writing*, 5(3), 281–296.

van Drempt, N., McCluskey, A., & Lannin, N. A. (2011). Handwriting in healthy people aged 65 years and over. *Australian Occupational Therapy Journal*, 58(4), 276–286. doi:10.1111/j.1440-1630.2011.00923.x.

Van Galen, G. P. (1991). Handwriting: Issues for a psychomotor theory. *Human Movement Science*, 10(2–3), 165–191.

van Hoorn, J. F., Maathuis, C. G. B., Peters, L. H. J., & Hadders-Algra, M. (2010a). Handwriting, visuomotor integration, and neurological condition at school age. *Developmental Medicine and Child Neurology*, 52(10), 941–947. doi:10.1111/j.1469-8749.2010.03715.x.

van Hoorn, J. F., Maathuis, C. G. B., Peters, L. H. J., & Hadders-Algra, M. (2010b). Handwriting, visuomotor integration, and neurological condition at school age. *Developmental Medicine and Child Neurology*, 52(10), 941–947. doi:10.1111/j.1469-8749.2010.03715.x.

Walker, L., & Henneberg, M. (2007). Writing with the non-dominant hand: Cross-handedness trainability in adult individuals. *Laterality*, 12(2), 121–130. doi:10.1080/13576500600989665.

Walton, J. (1997). Handwriting changes due to aging and Parkinson's syndrome. *Forensic Science International*, 88(3), 197–214.

Weintraub, N., Drory-Asayag, A., Dekel, R., et al. (2007). Developmental trends in handwriting performance among middle school children. *OTJR - Occupation Participation and Health*, 27(3), 104–112.

Wing, A. M., & Nimmo-Smith, I. (1987). The variability of cursive handwriting measure defined along a continuum: Letter specificity. *Journal of the Forensic Science Society*, 27(5), 297–306.

Yan, J. H., Rountree, S., Massman, P., et al. (2008). Alzheimer's disease and mild cognitive impairment deteriorate fine movement control. *Journal of Psychiatric Research*, 42(14), 1203–1212. doi:10.1016/j.jpsychires.2008.01.006.

Yan, Z., & Fischer, K. (2002). Always under construction – dynamic variations in adult cognitive microdevelopment. *Human Development*, 45(3), 141–160.

Yancosek, K. E., & Mullineaux, D. R. (2011). Stability of handwriting performance following injury-induced hand-dominance transfer in adults: A pilot study. *Journal of Rehabilitation Research and Development*, 48(1), 59–68. doi:10.1682/JRRD.2010.04.0074.

3
Signature Examination

3.1 Introduction

Signatures are a special kind of handwriting for a number of very important reasons. A signature is a way for a person to endorse the content of a document and this therefore goes beyond the creating of the content itself and means that a person is agreeing with that content. The most obvious example would be a cheque where the date, payee and amounts can be written by a third party, but it is the signature that is the component that effectively authorises the transfer of funds from the account. It is for this reason that the signature on a document is of particular relevance in many forensic cases.

Signatures can come in a wide variety of forms ranging from simple to complex, from legible to stylised (with few or no recognisable letterforms) and from full name to very shortened. A person's signature is, for some writers, their most frequently produced writing and is perhaps their most practised and automatic writing. As a result, signatures are often fluent even if other writing is less so, to the point where those who would be regarded as unable to write can at least sign their name.

Because of the significance attached to signatures, they are the primary target of simulation (copying by forgery) – far more so than normal handwriting. For this reason, as we shall see in Section 3.6 of this chapter when we consider how to interpret findings, the handwriting expert will have several alternatives to consider including the possibility that it is a genuine signature, a simulated copy of a genuine signature or a non-simulated version.

The production of signatures is physiologically similar to handwriting production as described in Chapter 2. The fluency and speed with which most people are able to execute their signature suggests that the motor plan is highly learned and automated. Since some writers have no recognisable

Foundations of Forensic Document Analysis: Theory and Practice, First Edition. Michael Allen.
© 2016 John Wiley & Sons, Ltd. Published 2016 by John Wiley & Sons, Ltd.
Companion Website: www.wiley.com/go/allen/forensicanalysis

letterforms in their signature, and given that there is no language input as such (other than perhaps spelling), the cognitive paths that initiate the movements for signatures are likely to be different in some respects to those associated with normal text.

Signatures show natural variation just as handwriting does. For many people a signature will be their most frequently executed written product and so might be expected to show strong similarity from one occasion to another. However, this is not necessarily the case as people vary in the consistency that their signatures show from one occasion to another. No two pieces of handwriting or signatures will ever be identical, but might it be possible that two signatures are so similar that they could be misidentified as one having been copied from the other?

The copying of signatures, whether it be freehand or by a tracing process, is itself imperfect, depending to some extent on the skill of the person doing the copying and the materials available. The penmanship of forgers has been examined (Dewhurst et al., 2008) and shown to be a factor, with skilled writers (calligraphers) better able to produce simulated signatures that cause problems for document examiners.

Given that signatures may not contain any recognisable letters, how is it possible to examine them at all? The reason is that signature comparison (indeed any handwriting comparison) is in reality a sophisticated pattern comparison process of a product of the human mind. The key point is that the comparison must be made on a like-with-like basis. In normal handwriting, the letters have to be identifiable so as to ensure that a like-with-like comparison is being made – the fact that the letter is an **A** or **B** or **C** is essentially immaterial. Hence, it is possible to compare signatures that are unreadable or indeed in a foreign script providing it is possible to be sure that they are purporting to be the same thing.

As a result, a master signature will not be identical to the copied signature derived from it. The degree of difference between the copy signature and a coincidentally similar genuine signature therefore becomes a theoretical possibility. The degree of similarity of just the height and length of signatures from the same writer was assessed by Evett and Totty, and the results provide evidence for expecting discernible variation to occur between genuine signatures (Evett & Totty, 1985). Indeed the authors found that over time the dimensions of signatures could vary, reinforcing the need to seek contemporary specimens whenever possible. In addition, traced signatures are by their very nature drawn rather than fluently written and hence the fluency is likely to be a key feature in discriminating between two coincidentally similar genuine signatures or a genuine signature and a tracing from it. The experienced document examiner should be able to distinguish between the various possible scenarios, and if there is uncertainty this will be reflected in the confidence with which a conclusion is expressed.

The expertise of forensic examiners is probably most tested by signature examinations due to the small amounts of writing involved and the willingness of fraudsters to try to perfect a simulation for whatever gain they have in mind. The capability of experts to reach a correct opinion is therefore nowhere more sharply focused than in signature examinations, where a correct opinion is that which is not only factually correct but also has the correct strength of opinion in terms of the available evidence (including an inconclusive opinion where the evidence does not support any view reliably).

3.2 The development of signatures

The factors that writers incorporate into their signature and how the decisions are made as to its form have received virtually no academic research. For many people the initial impetus to develop a signature will arise in their late teens or early 20s as they need to make decisions and transactions away from their parents and guardians, perhaps in education or in various dealings relating to property or finance. It is likely that most people will experiment with alternative forms of signature and settle on one that they like, because it is easy to write or pleasing aesthetically or for some other reason. However, it is also likely that the initial form may undergo some changes over time, perhaps major revision to begin with, but eventually settling into a form that becomes the highly automated signature that will remain for much of adult life. Signing one's name is something that some people will do much more than others, often depending on one's job. Frequent signing may lead to a person simplifying and/or shortening their signature to facilitate speed of execution. This may affect at least obvious properties, such as the size of the signature which can vary over time.

One obvious cause of a signature change is marriage, if one or other person takes the surname of their spouse. This requires the re-invention of a signature in a process that is presumably not unlike that when first a signature is created in adolescence (unless, by some unlikely event, there is no change due to coincidentally having the same surname).

One special example of the signature is the autograph used by celebrities. It is again a matter of the individual devising an autograph that suits their purpose and there may not necessarily be an obvious connection between an autograph and course-of-business signature of a celebrity. Because such signatures have a commercial value, there is a market for the buying and selling of autographs, and for this reason simulated autographs may be encountered by the forensic document examiner.

For the most part signatures, once their form has been finalised to the writer's satisfaction, will remain reasonably consistent over long periods of time. Indeed, the ability to write a signature is particularly resistant to the effects of age and incapacity that may occur later in life. This may be for a variety of reasons, including the automated nature of the process and also the personal significance that people attach to being able to sign their name.

Thus, the dynamics of signature development are similar in general terms to handwriting, except that the 'learning' phase occurs much later, typically in the teens, when normal handwriting has usually been mastered as a skill.

Signature writing is for many people a highly learned and automated skill. It was noted in Chapter 2 that such highly learned skills are difficult to copy by others attempting to adopt the relevant pen movements at the appropriate speed. Conversely, altering a signature to disguise it is difficult as the automatic movements are hard to suppress without losing natural fluency and appearance.

While a developed signature will be used by someone for many years, with often relatively little change, there are circumstances in which the signature can be affected, producing changes that require the document examiner's expertise to interpret what has caused the differences.

3.2.1   External influences: alcohol, infirmity and old age

In Chapter 2 a number of factors that can affect handwriting in general were discussed and these, of course, equally apply to signatures. For example, alcohol is likely to be a frequent external influence on handwriting and signature production. These effects are another reason why computer recognition of signatures is a difficult area. However, if it is known that the true signatory is drunk then automated systems can detect changes in the signature, such as lighter pen pressure and faster writing speed, and infer the possibility that the changes are due to intoxication (Shin & Okuyama, 2014).

Many of the factors that influence handwriting production in the infirm and elderly will also of course have the potential to affect signature execution. Because of the social and personal significance of the signature, even for those who find handwriting difficult, the production of a signature remains a matter of personal pride and it is common to see elderly people retouching their signature to make it 'look right'. The signature is nonetheless often the most highly practised handwriting movement and it may be particularly resistant by virtue of its automatic production to showing the effects that appear in everyday handwriting.

In general, the factors that affect handwriting and are discussed in detail in Chapter 2 will also have the potential to affect the appearance of the signature. However, it is possible that the interaction between the cognitive and motor aspects of normal handwriting are changed somewhat due to the minimal amount of thought that has to go into writing something as familiar as one's signature.

3.2.2 Guided hand signatures

If a person is incapacitated, for example due to ill health, then it may be allowable for them to be assisted by another person should they need to sign their name. It may be appropriate to query both their mental capacity to understand what they are signing and their physical capacity to execute the signature. The mental capacity to understand what they are doing is clearly outside the handwriting expert's remit. However, the effects on a signature that guidance from another person may lead to are legitimate areas for assessment by the handwriting expert.

Guided hand signature cases are rare. One of the key aspects to guided hand signatures is the extent of the assistance provided and the capacity of the true signatory to write their own signature (Sellers, 1962). In general, the greater the capacity of the true signatory to write, the less assistance that will need to be given (often just requiring support of the writing arm, for example, with no movement contributed by the assistant) and therefore the resulting guided hand signature will tend to look like a normal genuine signature. However, if the true signatory is severely incapacitated then the assistance will necessarily need to be greater and the true signatory may contribute little towards the movement of the pen, so that the formation of the signature will correspondingly be more influenced by the person doing the guiding. This will tend to produce a signature that has much less similarity to the true signatory's signature. If the input is fairly even, then the resulting signature may take on a mixture of the true signatory's handwriting features and those of the guide, an outcome that is extremely difficult to predict in advance. Guided hand signatures therefore display some often unexpectedly marked departures from the specimens due to the 'one off' interaction between the guider and the guided against a background of an otherwise fairly 'normal' looking signature. This tends to contrast with simulated signatures in which the forger attempts to minimise any differences with the genuine signature.

3.2.3 Signatures in blind people

Handwriting for blind or visually impaired people is extremely difficult, but fortunately the development of computer technology has enabled written communication. However, signing one's name is still a desirable skill to acquire and various devices have been created to assist with this, using specially modified pens that are held in a stand so that they maintain contact with the paper, and with tactile, kinaesthetic (sense of force on the body) and audio feedback in the learning process replacing visual feedback (Plimmer et al., 2011). The social acceptability of normal signatures may also be reflected on documents such as job applications, in which the inability to sign 'conventionally' may bias a potential employer's view of a candidate's capability.

3.3 Simulating signatures

There are a number of methods of simulating signatures. By far the most commonly encountered in casework is a freehand simulation, whereby the forger attempts to reproduce, without any aids, the signature of another person usually with reference to at least one sample of that person's signature. In many instances it is possible for the sample signature to be visible at the time that the simulation is written. Of course, this may not be possible in all circumstances, such as when signing in front of a witness in a bank or lawyer's office; in these situation forgers have to rely on their memory to recall what the signature looks like.

Copying the signature of another person is not easy as the forger will have their own handwriting features that will need to be suppressed, and at the same time the handwriting movements to produce the simulated signature have to be adopted while maintaining appropriate fluency throughout.

The ease with which a target signature can be copied will inevitably be determined in part by the complexity of that signature. A very simple signature is likely to be more accurately copied than a complex one. The complexity of the target signature is determined by a variety of factors such as its length, the overlapping pen-lines, the unusual formations of letters, the absence of recognisable letterforms and the presence of unusual shapes of curves and lines in their place and so on.

Whatever the nature of the target signature, the handwriting skill of the forger is another important aspect of the outcome of the simulation process. A person that cannot write skilfully will not be able to produce a fluent copy of a skilful writer's signature. It is not surprising that skilful forgers are often skilful penmen that also have a good eye for detail (Dewhurst et al., 2008).

Simulated signatures need to reproduce all elements of the target signature as closely as possible from the form to its proportions and its fluency (Figure 3.1). Simulations tend to fail more for reasons of lack of fluency, reflecting the forger's desire to make the signature appear as pictorially similar as possible. This has been confirmed as being true for other handwriting systems (for example, see Al-Musa Alkahtani and Platt (2010) for Arabic signatures).

Tracing signatures by various means are occasionally encountered in casework. A slight indentation in the paper surface is used as a guideline (for example, using tracing paper as an intermediate) and can be detected by close examination revealing the indented guideline running alongside the inked

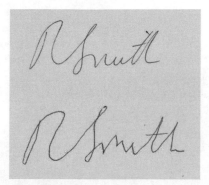

Figure 3.1 The upper signature has a smooth pen line with variation in pen pressure. The lower signature is a freehand simulation showing a shaky pen line and a 'drawn' appearance.

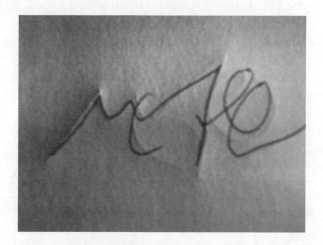

Figure 3.2 The tracing lines are close to, but not exactly overwritten by, the ink line.

signature at the points where the inking in does not follow exactly the guideline (Figure 3.2).

A genuine signature can be scanned and the signature printed out onto a document. Microscopy will show that a computer printer rather than a pen has been used. If the computer-printed signature is then inked in to mask this, the result is often very clumsy (Figure 3.3).

A so-called window tracing can be effected by placing the document that is to bear the simulation on top of a document bearing a genuine signature and illuminating them together from behind. The forger then produces the simulation by following the genuine signature that shows through. The simulation produced is usually of poor fluency and may well be incorrectly constructed since this process may only produce a pictorially similar simulation.

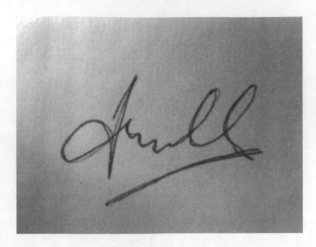

Figure 3.3   A scanned and printed signature overwritten in ink.

Any simulation based on a tracing or image-copying process can potentially be linked to the genuine (master) signature from which it is derived by overlaying the two signatures and finding them to be so similar that they cannot have been independently produced. (See Evett and Totty (1985) for a discussion of how similar two genuine signatures can be.)

One type of signature that is encountered in some parts of the world is the seal. This typically shows a signature that has been etched onto a wooden, plastic or metal substrate (see Box 3.1)

Box 3.1 Examination of signature seals

Seals are a means of rapidly applying a form of signature to a document, a practice that is widely accepted in many parts of the world as a means of authenticating a document (Lee et al., 2012). The seal may be made from various materials and the method of production of both genuine and counterfeit seals has become more sophisticated with the use of computer-aided manufacturing. The incidence of forged seal marks has risen in line with the availability of improved methods of counterfeit seal production.

Seals are a form of stampmark (see Chapter 5, Section 5.3.2). The method of forensic examination is therefore similar but the importance of the seal as a sign of authentication makes it even more significant. Indeed, some authorities require that genuine seals be registered and only permit the use of authorised seals. This highlights the importance of controlling access to the seals themselves so that counterfeit seals cannot be made as copies. But there is also the possibility of creating a counterfeit seal derived from a genuine seal impression on a document.

The improvement in the technology of counterfeit seal production has led to an increase in the number of forged seal marks, but has also assisted the forensic expert in ways of identifying forgeries. The essential task of showing that a seal mark is forged is to demonstrate that the questioned mark could not have been produced by the genuine seal. Genuine seal marks will show a range of variation in the marks caused by the relevant factors, including the amount of ink on the seal when applied, the pressure applied, the evenness of the pressure and the nature of the paper surface and its ink receptivity (with some papers showing the ink bleeding into the paper, for example).

Use of image processing software can compare specimen seal marks with that in question to see whether or not the images are similar or otherwise (Lee et al., 2012). Essentially this amounts to overlaying the images of the genuine and suspect seal marks to see how closely they correspond. If one or other seal mark crosses other text, then this needs to be removed from the image using the image software. Further, because each seal image is unique depending on the various factors mentioned above, no one specimen can be representative. One way to try to overcome this is to use image software to take an average from a number of specimen seal marks so that any minor inconsistencies caused, for example, by a lack of ink in part of one seal mark are compensated by other specimens that do not show that lack of ink.

By comparing the images of genuine and questioned seal marks and using statistical methods to assess the degree of similarity of pixel (picture elements) alignment between the images on the basis of various mathematical functions, it is possible to determine the likelihood that a suspect seal mark is genuine or otherwise.

3.4 Computer-based recognition of signatures

Identifying a person has many important functions in society. There are many ways in which a person's identity can be confirmed, ranging from those who know the person to other means such as documentation (a passport for example). In this context, identification is the process of determining who someone is (comparing one from many, for example by examining photographs of a set of people) whereas verification confirms a person's identity (comparing one against one, for example comparing someone with the passport photograph) and such comparisons often involve the use of biometrics. Biometrics are, as their name suggests, ways of differentiating between people using various measures. These measures can be of two types. Physiological measures, such as fingerprints or iris eye patterns, measure aspects of the body as a physical object. Behavioural biometrics measure features caused by the body moving, such as how one walks (gait pattern), speech patterns or signature writing. As people will vary in almost any behavioural activity, biometrics that can capture this variability have the potential to assist in identification with all the ramifications that this has in a modern society.

The use of signatures as biometrics has been, and continues to be, extensively researched. Automatic signature analysis has been used in the banking industry and its use in other aspects of everyday security is under constant review. The frequency with which signatures are used in all kinds of social and financial transactions serves only to emphasise their importance. Crucially, it is almost always the case that the person who may be 'accepting' the signature (such as a shop keeper) is not trained sufficiently to be able to reliably assess a signature's authenticity. For this reason, a considerable amount of effort has gone into using computers to assess whether a signature is genuine or not.

There are two types of feature that machines can analyse. Some features can be derived from the static image of the completed signature, such as its size and the geometrical conformations of various elements such as loop shapes. The second kind are dynamic features such as the speed of pen movement and pen pressure. Dynamic features can only be measured accurately using the appropriate technology, namely a digitising tablet (see Box 2.2 in Chapter 2). Technological improvements to these devices have been mirrored to some extent by the many different ways in which the information attained is processed using various algorithms that extract from the data key comparison parameters. For example, the simple maximum dimensions could be measured or the velocity of pen movement could be measured or the number of acceleration and decelerations could be counted. Deciding which parameters to use and how to incorporate them into an algorithm that minimises errors is itself a key factor in the success of these systems (Wilkin & Ooi Shih Yin, 2011).

Such automated systems of signature comparison can produce two types of error. Type I errors are false rejections (where a signature is assessed as being not genuine when in fact it is genuine) and type II errors are false acceptances (where a signature is deemed to be genuine when in fact it is not genuine). Verification devices (note that to verify a person's signature requires that they have previously recorded their signature one or more times for comparison purposes) will show both error types and such errors are more or less likely to occur depending upon the nature of the signatures being studied. For example, if specimen (previously recorded) and questioned (the signature being verified) signatures are all naturally written then the error rates are lower, but if a questioned signature is disguised it may be wrongly deemed to be not genuine when in fact it is (type I error) or a skilful simulation may be deemed to be genuine when it is not (type II error). Genuine signatures that are fairly simple in formation and consistent may lead to many correct verifications with few false rejections. Similarly, if forged signatures are very crude these may be readily rejected with few false acceptances. However, this assumes a fairly naïve level of expectation from real-world situations where some people naturally have very variable signatures and some forgers do make considerable efforts to perfect simulated signatures. Such situations are a much greater challenge to automated systems and even a relatively low level of improvement and motivation by the forger can cause false acceptance of forgeries as genuine signatures (Ballard et al., 2007).

Signature variability must be accounted for in automated systems of signature verification, but variability itself varies from person to person. In addition, increased variability is often found in the signatures of older people due to general loss of motor control together with any relevant medical conditions. Thus age and health are particular factors that such systems may need to consider (Guest, 2006), factors that the forensic expert is trained to routinely consider when relevant.

Not only can such devices measure what is happening during the writing process, they are also capable of measuring the movement and time that the pen is not writing, in other words when the pen is in the air. It has been shown that the writer's habits also apply to the non-writing component as the pen moves from one part of the writing to the next. This will have particular value in text production where there are more such non-writing movements, but if a signature has breaks in it these too may be a characteristic (Sesa-Nogueras et al., 2012).

Both the dynamic and static dimensions of signature production are potentially legitimate sources of (imperfect) information about a person's identity. The amount of information available from the static image is significantly less and this inevitably leads to a much larger error rate in assessing signature authenticity, whereas the dynamic information leads to a smaller error rate (Kovari & Charaf, 2013).

However, global error rates do not show the level of difficulty in any particular comparison. Signature complexity, the ability of writers to disguise their own signatures or copy the signatures of others may all contribute to greater error rates in verification systems. Computers cannot readily account for the human dimensions of cunning and skill, which is where the forensic document examiner's experience of casework is of greatest value. Nonetheless, the evaluation of output from an automated (biometric) system with associated false rejection and false acceptance rates can be mapped onto a Bayesian approach (see Section 2.9.2 of Chapter 2) of evidence assessment (based on alternative hypotheses) with the use of mathematical manipulation (Gonzalez-Rodriguez et al., 2005).

Given the desire to minimise errors, one possibility is to use more than one biometric approach. For example, it is possible to record and measure pen grip, which could give yet more information about the writer. The way that a person holds the writing implement itself may be fairly characteristic (although very unlikely to be unique). There are a number of general ways of holding a pen (Schneck & Henderson, 1990). Measuring the relative amounts of contact between the writer and the writing implement (using a pen specially adapted and fitted with pressure sensors) adds another layer of information that can be derived from the signing process (Ghali et al., 2013). This grip pattern will be a reflection of how much pressure the fingers and hand place at various points around and along the barrel of the implement, a pattern that will show some variability depending on the physical properties of the implement, such as its diameter and shape.

A second possibility would be to use a signature together with speech recognition. Research has suggested that the signature and spoken name together provide more information than either on their own (Humm et al., 2009). To make an effective forgery would thus require imitation of the voice as well as the handwriting by the impostor. The advantage of speech verification is that it can occur at essentially the same timescale as the signing process.

The advanced devices used in handwriting research should not be confused with the devices used by delivery services, for example, where receipt of goods is endorsed by signing at the front door. Such devices are not intended to be used in the research laboratory but are a convenient way of recording signatures, albeit the forensic information available from such devices is limited.

In summary, the investigation into the mechanics of handwriting and the use of signatures as a biometric have reinforced the considerable scope that handwriting and signatures have for distinguishing between people or, alternatively, confirming a person's identity. However, the hardware and software (algorithms) used have yet to replace the forensic document examiner, whose experience at interpreting the evidence has not been improved upon (see Box 3.2).

Box 3.2 Expertise of forensic document examiners

Since a signature is often such an important component of a document, there is an issue about who should be able to authenticate a signature. For example, it would seem reasonable, on the face of it, for someone to be able to say whether or not a signature in their own name is genuine or not. Then that could perhaps be extended to identifying the signatures of spouses, family members or indeed anyone whose signature may be familiar. However, this is a far from satisfactory idea since, for example, people often do not recall actually signing a document but claim to recognise their signature from its appearance. Memory is not always accurate, especially in the more elderly, and of course people may have a vested interest in saying whether a signature is theirs or not. The document examiner, therefore, not only brings expertise to the examination but also, crucially, impartiality.

This also begs the question of just what it is that makes a witness an expert witness. It is a widely misunderstood idea that an expert witness is someone who is a uniquely knowledgeable world authority on a subject. This is not the case. In those jurisdictions that have attempted to identify what qualifies someone to be an expert witness, the main requirement is that an expert witness should have knowledge, experience and expertise above and beyond that which a lay person might reasonably be expected to have in that discipline.

It is right that any forensic speciality should be able to show that the methods used and the conclusions drawn are reliable in principle, being based on a significant body of widely accepted and published knowledge (as distinct from the competence of individual experts to apply the knowledge and theories that underpin the speciality). Traditionally, this has not always happened as much as it should and the robustness of the knowledge has not been vigorously challenged.

In more recent times, the claims of forensic science have become increasingly questioned across all disciplines (for example, The Law Commission in England and Wales (2011) and National Research Council (2009) in the USA). In questioned documents, the spotlight has fallen particularly on the examination of signatures since this is arguably one of the hardest elements of the expert's job. The focus has been on a number of elements of the expert's role:

- Are document examiners in fact more accurate than lay people at identifying handwriting and, in particular signatures? One of the earliest papers to address this question was by Kam and colleagues. Their results showed that document examiners are indeed significantly better at coming to the correct conclusion than are lay people (Kam et al., 2001).

- What in fact do document examiners bring to their speciality that lay persons do not? What do experts look at, how do they reach their conclusions? The ways in which experts observe and assimilate information about signatures has been studied, revealing shifts of focus shown by the eye movement in document examiners. This indicates that the expert is seeking multiple pieces of information from the signatures being examined (rather than just one overriding piece of evidence). The wide-ranging attention to different aspects of a signature implies that a variety of pieces of evidence are being focused on, consistent with the different potential explanations that the expert will be considering for their findings (Dyer et al., 2006).

- What types of cases cause experts the most difficulty? Bird and colleagues found that handwriting experts were very good at determining whether a signature was naturally written or not in comparison to specimen signatures. However, experts were less reliable when it came to determining the *cause* of the unnatural signature, that is distinguishing between simulations (written by someone other than the true signatory but attempting to copy the true signatory's signature) and disguised signatures (written by the true signatory but attempting to alter their signature) (Bird et al., 2010).

- Are experts influenced by other external factors when reaching conclusions? The idea that experts might be influenced by case circumstances, other information given to them by an investigator for instance (so called cognitive bias), or even the financial payment for their services, has been investigated. In questioned documents, the idea that handwriting experts' opinions might be influenced by extrinsic inducements was not supported (Dewhurst et al., 2014).

3.5   The forensic examination of signatures

The basis of the forensic comparison process is essentially the same as that described for handwriting comparisons. Generally speaking, obtaining specimen signatures is not a problem as few people are unable to produce some kind of signature. Even those who have not learned to write, for whatever reason, can generally write their signature, although such signatures are often relatively simple in their formation and may not be very fluently written.

The fact that signatures can be modified over time due to a variety of reasons makes it important that specimens are as contemporary as possible to the disputed signature. The number of specimen signatures needed varies from case to case but typically about 12 is a good starting point from documents signed in the course of everyday life. Some people do not have cause to sign their names very often and it may be necessary to ask for specimen signatures to be supplied at request. The limitation of request specimen signatures is similar to that for normal handwriting, because requested signatures can only provide a snapshot of the range of variation to be found in a person's signature. With request specimens, the possibility of deliberate disguise always has to be considered, and this is even more likely to happen with signatures that can be changed relatively easily. However, disguise is not always very subtle and is often readily apparent due to loss of fluency, loss of consistency and, if available, a lack of similarity to any non-request signatures. Disguise of signatures, while relatively simple to do at the gross level, is much more difficult to do at a subtle level since the signing process is so automated that making small changes is more difficult than a complete transformation. When asked to make relatively subtle adjustments to their signature with the intention of later denying authorship, most people find it very difficult to achieve because of the automatic nature with which signatures are usually written. Any interruption caused by the intended changes lead to disruption of the motor pattern which is reflected in poor execution.

Making a comparison between the questioned signatures and specimens is very similar to that described for handwriting in the previous chapter. All relevant observations must be recorded, such as the structure, the variation, the proportions and the fluency, and these are compared between the questioned and specimen signatures. Because signing is just as prone to natural variation as handwriting is, there will always be some features that can be matched and others that cannot. It is the task of the expert to interpret the meaning of the findings and reach a safe and justified conclusion based on interpretation of all of the observations.

3.6 Interpreting findings in signature cases

Most of the features that the handwriting expert examines in signature cases are static features of shape, proportion and slope. Measurements of pen speed are not possible from the static image of the signature, but some dynamic aspects of signature production can be inferred. Just as with handwriting examinations, the speed of pen movement and the pressure applied to the writing implement can be inferred from the pen line. Pen pressure and pen speed are important diagnostic features in all signature cases since a forger may not write at the same speed or with the same pressure as the true signatory. Likewise, a person attempting to alter their signature deliberately may change the speed or pressure as they concentrate on making the changes.

The experience of the expert is crucial in assessing which explanation best fits the observations in a particular signature case. As with handwriting examinations, alternative explanations must be considered. A detailed Bayesian approach to a signature case is reported by Biedermann et al. (2012).

The various explanations for findings in relation to the authorship of a questioned signature are as follows, although not all possibilities may be relevant in all cases (Figure 3.4).

1. *A genuine signature written in normal circumstances* – typically while seated at a table. Normal, genuine signatures usually lie within the range of variation to be found in the specimen signatures and will show a similar fluency when compared to the specimens.

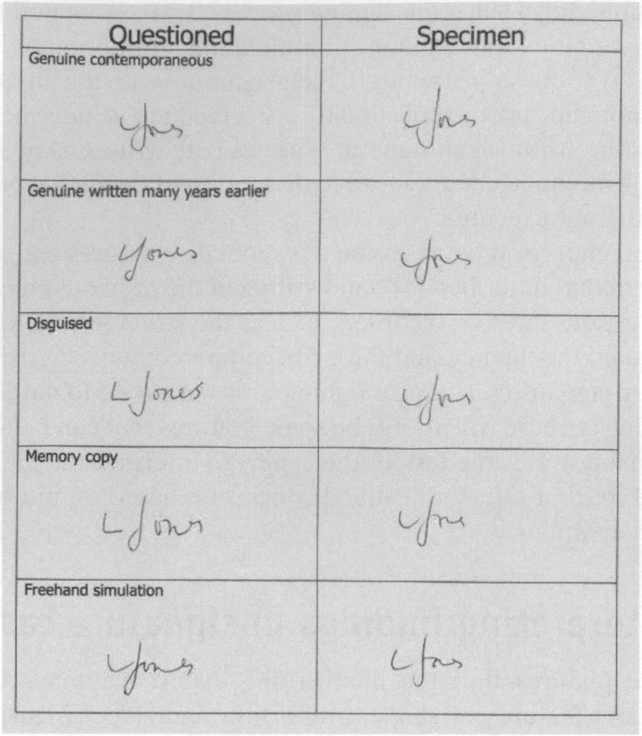

Figure 3.4 Five naturally written specimen signatures compared to (i) a genuine signature written at about the same time; (ii) a genuine signature written many years earlier; (iii) a disguised signature written by the true signatory; (iv) a memory copy; (v) a freehand simulation.

2. *A genuine signature written at a different time* to the specimens with differences attributable to changes in the signature over time. If there is a known significant time gap between the specimen and questioned signatures, especially when it involves young, typically teenage, or older people, then due caution must be used to take account of the possibility of experimental and developmental changes in the young and loss of pen control in the elderly.

3. *A genuine signature written in unusual circumstances* but with no intention to alter it (for example, written while drunk, or using an unusual writing implement or standing and supporting paper on an infirm surface). If it is known that a signature was written in unusual circumstances, then it may be possible to use this information to anticipate what effect it might have on a signature. For example, as noted in Section 3.2.1, alcohol tends to lead to a relaxation of movement and signatures reflect this by being larger and tending towards a more scribbled appearance, but the fundamental structure usually is kept.

4. *A genuine but disguised signature* that has been intentionally changed or a simulation of a genuine signature. In casework, this distinction is often the most crucial. Deliberate disguise where the writer intends to deny their signature at a later time (for instance due to not having sufficient funds to cover a financial commitment) can vary in extent from just a minor alteration, such as using a middle initial when it is usually absent, writing a first name in full rather than using initials or adding an underline, to changing some letterforms. Changes can be to individual letters or can be more global, such as a change of slope. For most writers for whom writing a signature is automatic, such changes lead to significant disruption to the fluency and most people can only modify a small number of features of their signature – changing the appearance of each component of the signature is extremely difficult to achieve in most cases. The nature of the disguise is also an important factor; counter-intuitively, the more subtle changes are more difficult to achieve than the gross, obvious changes since the former require more careful thought whereas the latter can involve a single major change such as writing in capital letters. The need for subtle change is sometimes referred to as autoforgery to distinguish it from very obvious differences where the resemblance to a usual signature is minimal. The need for subtle change is greater if the person accepting the signature has any basis for a comparison with a genuine signature (such as on a cheque guarantee card) such that a gross deviation would be obvious and call the authenticity of the signature into immediate doubt and non-acceptance.

If the questioned signature has been disguised but the specimens are natural, then typically there is at least some degree of similarity between the questioned and specimen signatures but also differences. The problem for the expert is that this general description also applies when the questioned signature is a simulated copy written by some other person. The nature of each individual difference and similarity must then be assessed in terms of how closely it matches the specimens, not only in terms of form and structure but also fluency.

Bird and colleagues showed that experts do indeed have most difficulty distinguishing between, on the one hand, genuine but disguised signatures written by the true signatory and, on the other hand, simulated signatures written by some other person attempting to reproduce the appearance of the true signatory's signature (Bird et al., 2010). The reason is that the resulting differences may appear similar in that in both cases there is usually a loss of fluency and also some difference in form or structure which are minimised to improve acceptability. The key point is that a forger is attempting to minimise differences whereas the disguiser is attempting to have as much difference from their normal signature as they believe will be accepted and not rejected. In addition, if the signature is complex, the forger may simply construct it incorrectly, whereas as noted above, the pen movements are so highly automated for the true writer that these remain similar even when introducing changes to the appearance of characters.

The authorship of a simulated, forged signature is almost always impossible to determine (Hilton, 1952). The reason is that the natural handwriting characteristics of the forger are suppressed as they attempt to adopt handwriting features of the person whose signature they are copying. One exception is where at least parts of the forger's name and that of the target signature are shared, for example where the surname is shared. In such circumstances, there may be some evidence that parts of the questioned signature are more similar to the forger's natural handwriting characteristics and differ from the natural signature of the person whose signature has been copied.

5. *A memory copy*. The ability of someone to copy a signature based on recall will depend in part on the circumstances. Husbands and wives may become very familiar with each other's signature, for example, and indeed may regularly 'sign for each other' which goes unchallenged unless and until there is a marital dispute! However, the recall is not usually as good as believed by those concerned and distinguishing the true signature from that of the frequent copier is often not difficult.

6. *A genuine signature of someone using more than one style of signature*. It may be that the different forms share certain features or they may be completely unrelated.

7. *An accidental* caused by a one off disturbance to the normal process of signing. Such signatures usually appear fluent for the most part and similar to the specimen signatures, but where the disruption to the signature occurs it is temporary as the writer regains the pattern of movement needed to complete the signature.

8. *A guided hand signature*. For a detailed discussion see Section 3.2.2.

9. *A made up signature* written by someone else with no knowledge of, or attempt to simulate, what a genuine signature looks like. This is the one situation where it may be possible to indicate who wrote the non-genuine signature since the writer's own handwriting features may appear in the made up signature (Hilton, 1952).

Many documents are copied and the originals destroyed and the expert may have to do what they can based on often less than ideal quality copy documents. Physical evidence of tracing may well not be discernible from such documents and the fluency and structure of any complex overlapping pen lines may also be impossible to decipher. This can impose a severe limitation on what the expert can say in such cases and considerable caution may be needed before expressing an opinion on the authorship of a questioned signature shown on a copy document. Indeed, with the scanning and printing capabilities of modern technology, a signature that makes no attempt to be original but is shown by a copy document may well be a genuine signature that has been copied from elsewhere and added to a bogus document.

3.7 Note taking in signature cases

The notes that need to be made are inevitably very similar to those described in Chapter 2 for handwriting cases. The main difference is the need to consider very specifically the evidence for any relevant alternatives with the main points being to determine whether a questioned signature is genuine or not and, in particular, to distinguish between disguised genuine signatures and simulations. Any relevant information about the health or age of the person concerned should be explicitly mentioned and the influence this has on the final conclusion noted.

The adequacy, or otherwise, of the specimen signatures should be noted – are there enough of them and are they reasonably contemporary to the questioned signatures – crucial if the person is very ill, for example. The quality of copy documents supplied should also be noted and any details that cannot be discerned from the copy should be indicated as an area of uncertainty so that if an opinion has to be qualified it is clear why this is the case.

3.8 Reports in signature cases

The manner in which reports are written in cases involving signatures is similar to that described at the end of Chapter 2 for handwriting. For example, the limitations in a case need to be described so that reasons for a qualified opinion are made clear for the reader.

In handwriting cases the question of authorship usually revolves around the central question: was this piece of disputed handwriting written by the same person that wrote the specimen handwriting – yes or no. However, in signature cases this question is significantly modified in most instances as there is usually a need to specifically consider whether a disputed signature is either genuine or a simulation written by some other person attempting to copy a genuine signature of the true signatory. It is not so common for a questioned signature to be simply written by another person making no attempt whatsoever to copy some other person's signature.

For these reasons, the specific alternatives must be clearly stated in the report so that the findings of similarity and difference between a questioned and specimen signature can be considered in relation to them. If the conclusion is that a signature is genuine then that requires straightforward justification in the report, such as similar fluency, significant similarity in features and complex structure, all of which make simulation unlikely. However, if there is evidence of free-hand simulation (not by tracing of some kind), then identifying the author of the questioned signature is usually difficult or impossible and the reasons for this conclusion need to be briefly stated in the report by, for example, saying that when one person attempts to copy some else's signature they have to suppress their own handwriting habits and try to adopt those of the person whose signature they are copying – which inevitably changes their natural handwriting.

If a questioned signature is considered by the expert to be genuine but deliberately disguised, then the reasons for this need to be made clear especially in comparison to the possibility of simulation. Here, the *nature* of the differences will usually be the key issue and this needs to be clearly described so that the justification for the opinion is comprehensible to the non-expert.

Signature comparison: a worked example

In this section, an example of how to approach a case and make notes is demonstrated. It should be stressed that there are a number of different ways to make notes and the intention here is to show the kinds of issues that need to be considered and how these interrelate with the observation process leading to a conclusion.

Case circumstances

A business agreement between Mr R Smith and Mr V Murray regarding the purchase of shares in a company was drawn up. The contents of this agreement are now in dispute before the courts. In particular, Mr Smith says that the agreement put before the court by Mr Murray is not the one that he signed and that the signature in his (Mr Murray's) name that is on it is a forgery.

Purpose

To compare the questioned signature on the agreement with the specimen signatures supplied by Mr Murray with a view to determining whether or not he wrote it.

Items submitted

Item 1: Agreement (Figure 3.5)

Item 2: Specimen signatures of Mr Murray (Figure 3.6)

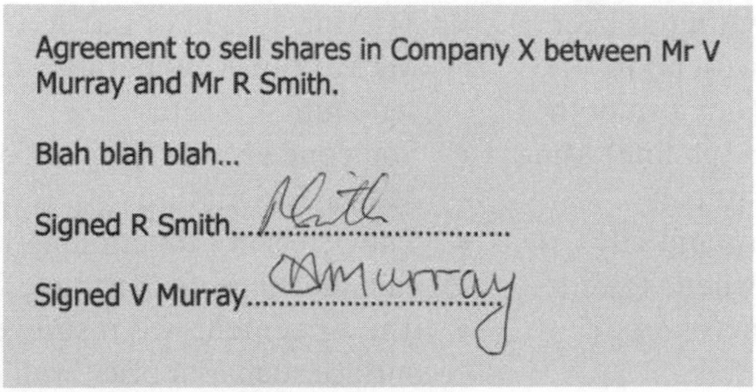

Agreement to sell shares in Company X between Mr V Murray and Mr R Smith.

Blah blah blah...

Signed R Smith.....................

Signed V Murray.....................

Figure 3.5   Worked example: Agreement.

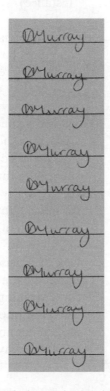

Figure 3.6   Worked example: Specimen signatures.

Case notes

Observations	Thoughts
Examination of the questioned signature shows that it has been written with poor fluency (not a smooth and even ink line) using a ballpoint pen (striations and oily deposit when viewed under microscope).	Reasons for poor fluency: • Mr Murray is not a very skilful writer. • Mr Murray is ill or old. • Mr Murray is deliberately changing his signature – disguise. • Someone else is trying to copy Mr Murray's signature. • The pen is not functioning very well (ink blockage, for example). • The agreement was resting on a rough surface such as a brick wall or an unstable support (writing whilst agreement balanced on one's knee for instance).
The specimen signatures are on a single sheet of paper written at request.	The specimen is not ideal because the signatures have been written on one occasion at request and for these reasons they cannot be fully representative. However, inspection of the specimen signatures shows them to be fluent, skilful and consistent, strongly suggesting that they are fairly representative of how Mr Murray signs his name. Any suggestion of disguise in the specimen signatures would be apparent through loss of fluency and lack of consistency. Overall, the material submitted is suitable for a meaningful comparison between the questioned signature on the agreement and the specimen signatures of Mr Murray.

Observations	Thoughts
Carefully examine the structure of questioned signature showing proportions and structure (particularly the path that the pen takes through the signature).	The questioned signature is relatively simple in its formation, which would enable a forger to determine the correct sequence of pen movements required. However, shapes of curves are distinctive and would be quite difficult to copy accurately. The reasonably distinctive appearance of the specimen and questioned signatures rules out any likelihood of a chance similarity – some other person *by chance* producing a signature that looks like Mr Murray's signature.
Carefully examine the structure of the specimen signatures showing proportions and structure (particularly the path that the pen takes through the signature). Note variations in the details.	The detailed examination confirms the initial appraisal that these are skilfully written signatures that show all the indications expected in normal, natural signatures – in particular there is no suggestion that Mr Murray has disguised his signature in the specimen provided.
Compare the detailed formation of the questioned signature with the specimen signatures of Mr Murray, noting any similarities and differences between them. (In the expert's opinion) the differences are significant the similarities are attributable to an attempt to make the questioned signature appear to be genuine.	The appearance of the questioned signature is similar to that of the specimen signatures and the proportions of letters differ from those in the specimens. Possible explanations: 1. Normal genuine signature – unlikely as specimens show him to be consistent and skilful when signing.

Observations	Thoughts
	2. Disguised signature written by Mr Murray but deliberately changing it – again unlikely because there is such a loss of fluency and the proportions differ.
	3. Forgery – the questioned signature shows all of the typical hallmarks associated with forged signatures, particularly the lack of fluency and the poor proportions despite an overall attempt to reproduce the pictorial appearance of Mr Murray's signature.
Summary	There is strong evidence that the questioned signature was not written by Mr Murray but rather is an attempt by some other person to copy his signature.

Report of Forensic Expert

Qualifications and experience ...

Scope of expertise ...

Items examined

I have examined the following items at the instruction of (the investigating authority). They were received at the laboratory on (dates).

Item 1: Agreement

Item 2: Specimen signatures of Mr Murray

Purpose

I have compared the questioned signature in the name of Mr Murray on item 1 with specimens of his signature, item 2, with a view to determining whether or not Mr Murray wrote the signature in his name on item 1.

Findings

The specimen signatures of Mr Murray have all been obtained on one occasion and cannot be fully representative of his signature. However, they are fluent and consistent and I have taken them to be fairly representative of his signature.

There is some pictorial similarity between the questioned signature and the specimen signatures of Mr Murray such that the questioned signature must either have been written by him or else by some other person making an attempt to copy his signature; a chance similarity can be excluded due to the distinctive nature of his signature.

The questioned signature has not been fluently written in contrast Mr Murray's specimen signatures which are skilfully written. The proportions and letter shapes of the specimen signatures are consistent from one to another and differ from those of the questioned signature. In my opinion, there is strong evidence that the questioned signature was not written by Mr Murray but rather is an attempt by some other person to copy his signature.

Summary

There is strong evidence that the signature in question was not written by Mr Murray but rather is an attempt by some other person to copy his signature.

References

Al-Musa Alkahtani, A., & Platt, A. W. G. (2010). A statistical study of the relative difficulty of freehand simulation of form, proportion, and line quality in Arabic signatures. *Science & Justice*, 50(2), 72–76.

Anonymous. (2011). *Expert Evidence in Criminal Proceedings in England and Wales.* (No. LC325). London: Law Commission.

Ballard, L., Lopresti, D., & Monrose, F. (2007). Forgery quality and its implications for behavioral biometric security. *Ieee Transactions on Systems Man and Cybernetics Part B-Cybernetics*, 37(5), 1107–1118. doi:10.1109/TSMCB.2007.903539

Biedermann, A., Voisard, R., & Taroni, F. (2012). Learning about Bayesian networks for forensic interpretation: An example based on the 'the problem of multiple propositions'. *Science & Justice*, 52(3), 191–198. doi:10.1016/j.scijus.2012.05.004

Bird, C., Found, B., Ballantyne, K., & Rogers, D. (2010). Forensic handwriting examiners' opinions on the process of production of disguised and simulated signatures. *Forensic Science International*, 195(1–3), 103–107. doi: 10.1016/j.forsciint.2009.12.001

Dewhurst, T. N., Found, B., Ballantyne, K. N., & Rogers, D. (2014). The effects of extrinsic motivation on signature authorship opinions in forensic signature blind trials. *Forensic Science International*, 236, 127–132. doi:10.1016/j.forsciint.2013.12.025

Dewhurst, T., Found, B., & Rogers, D. (2008). Are expert penmen better than lay people at producing simulations of a model signature? *Forensic Science International*, 180(1), 50–53. doi: 10.1016/j.forsciint.2008.06.009

Dyer, A. G., Found, B., & Rogers, D. (2006). Visual attention and expertise for forensic signature analysis. *Journal of Forensic Sciences*, 51(6), 1397–1404. doi:10.1111/j.1556-4029 .2006.00269.x ER

Evett, I. W., & Totty, R. N. (1985). A study of the variation in the dimensions of genuine signatures. *Journal of the Forensic Science Society*, 25(3), 207–215. doi:10.1016/S0015-7368(85)72393-6

Ghali, B., Thalanki Anantha, N., Chan, J., & Chau, T. (2013). Variability of grip kinetics during adult signature writing. *Plos One*, 8(5), e63216. Retrieved from 10.1371%2Fjournal.pone.0063216

Gonzalez-Rodriguez, J., Fierrez-Aguilar, J., Ramos-Castro, D., & Ortega-Garcia, J. (2005). Bayesian analysis of fingerprint, face and signature evidences with automatic biometric systems. *Forensic Science International*, 155(2–3), 126–140. doi:10.1016/j.forsciint.2004.11.007

Guest, R. (2006). Age dependency in handwritten dynamic signature verification systems. *Pattern Recognition Letters*, 27(10), 1098–1104. doi:10.1016/j.patrec.2005.12.008

Hilton, O. (1952). Can the forger be identified from his handwriting? *The Journal of Criminal Law, Criminology, and Police Science*, 43(4), 547–555. Retrieved from http://www.jstor.org/stable/1139367

Humm, A., Hennebert, J., & Ingold, R. (2009). Combined handwriting and speech modalities for user authentication. *Ieee Transactions on Systems Man and Cybernetics Part A-Systems and Humans*, 39(1), 25–35. doi:10.1109/TSMCA.2008.2007978

Kam, M., Gummadidala, K., Fielding, G., & Conn, R. (2001). Signature authentication by forensic document examiners. *Journal of Forensic Sciences*, 46(4), 884–888.

Kovari, B., & Charaf, H. (2013). A study on the consistency and significance of local features in off-line signature verification. *Pattern Recognition Letters*, 34(3), 247–255. doi:10.1016/j.patrec.2012.10.011

Lee, J., Kong, S. G., Lee, Y., et al. (2012). Forged seal detection based on the seal overlay metric. *Forensic Science International*, 214(1–3), 200–206. doi:10.1016/j.forsciint.2011.08.009

National Research Council. (2009). *Strengthening Forensic Science in the United States: A Path Forward*. Washington DC: The National Academies Press.

Plimmer, B., Reid, P., Blagojevic, R., et al. (2011). Signing on the tactile line: A multimodal system for teaching handwriting to blind children. *ACM Transactions on Computer-Human Interaction*, 18(3), 17. doi:10.1145/1993060.1993067

Schneck, C. M., & Henderson, A. (1990). Descriptive analysis of the developmental progression of grip position for pencil and crayon control in nondysfunctional children. *The American Journal of Occupational Therapy*, 44(10), 893–900.

Sellers, C. (1962). Assisted and guided signatures. *The Journal of Criminal Law, Criminology, and Police Science*, 53(2), 245–248. Retrieved from http://www.jstor.org/stable/1141089

Sesa-Nogueras, E., Faundez-Zanuy, M., & Mekyska, J. (2012). An information analysis of in-air and on-surface trajectories in online handwriting. *Cognitive Computation*, 4(2), 195–205. doi:10.1007/s12559-011-9119-y

Shin, J., & Okuyama, T. (2014). Detection of alcohol intoxication via online handwritten signature verification. *Pattern Recognition Letters*, 35:101–104. doi:10.1016/j.patrec.2012.07.016

Wilkin, T., & Ooi Shih Yin. (2011). State of the art: Signature verification system. Paper presented at the Information Assurance and Security (IAS), 2011 7th International Conference, 110–115. doi:10.1109/ISIAS.2011.6122804

4
Documents Produced Using Office Technology

4.1 Introduction

Having explored in depth the processes of writing and signing in Chapters 2 and 3, in this chapter the emphasis will be on the ways in which the written word is put on paper by means of mechanical devices. In order to understand how a forensic examination of documents produced with such devices is made, it is first necessary to understand the mechanisms of the machines themselves. The mechanisms together with the inks used dictate what the output looks like on paper. From this, it is possible to shed light on possible avenues of forensic evidence that can determine which kind of mechanism was involved in the production of a document and potentially which individual machine was responsible.

The underlying principles for examining machine-produced documents are essentially similar irrespective of the type of machine. The first step is to understand in general terms the manufacturing of the device. Ideally, all newly manufactured devices and their components should work perfectly and all be identical to one another, be they laser printers or fax machines or whatever. (Whether that is the case depends on the quality control systems in place as goods leave the factory.) As soon as machines start to be used, then wear and tear will start to play a part in the deterioration of that device. Since the use that devices receive will vary, the pattern of deterioration caused by wear and tear has the potential to make each machine uniquely identifiable providing there are ways to discern the effects of the changes from an examination of the documents produced from it. This is the single

Foundations of Forensic Document Analysis: Theory and Practice, First Edition. Michael Allen.
© 2016 John Wiley & Sons, Ltd. Published 2016 by John Wiley & Sons, Ltd.
Companion Website: www.wiley.com/go/allen/forensicanalysis

most important general principle in the identification of documents produced by machines.

In the not too distant past, machine-produced documents tended to be more frequently encountered in office and business settings as opposed to the domestic market, where such devices tended to be expensive and not needed in the days before the personal computer. It is true to say that quite a few homes did have a typewriter, for instance, but this was nowhere near as universal as the presence of the PC and associated printers and scanners is today.

During the transitional period from the typewriter to the computer printer (roughly speaking the 1980s and 1990s) computer printers started out being very expensive but increased demand and technological improvements led to a huge drop in price and made such machines commonplace and affordable to most. The transformation in less than a generation has been considerable and poses new challenges for the forensic document examiner.

4.2 Typewriters

The typewriter was invented in the late 1800s and its presence increased steadily in the business market into the 1980s, after which time there was a fairly rapid decline to the point where typewriters are now rarely encountered in casework. Rarely encountered, but just occasionally a typewriter features in a case and there remains the need for a document examiner to be able to examine the documents and, where relevant, the typewriter to interpret findings.

The first machines that were made were so-called typebar typewriters. These devices had the typeface placed on a series of about 40 typebars arranged in a basket-like configuration (Figure 4.1).

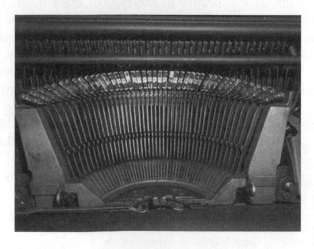

Figure 4.1   The arrangement of typebars.

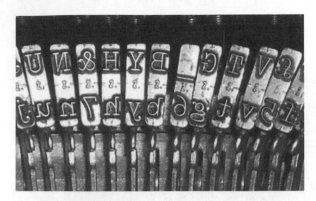

Figure 4.2 Two characters are present at the end of each typebar with the upper one accessed by using the shift mechanism (x3 approx.).

The typebars were made of metal. The ends of the typebars were fitted with metal pieces on which the typeface was present. Usually, each piece of metal had two characters present, such as the lower case (small form) and the upper case (capital form) of a given letter (Figure 4.2), or the various numerals and symbols which are largely retained on the modern computer keyboard.

The shapes of the various letters, numerals and other characters comprise the font style. Certain fonts, such as Times New Roman, were widely used and became almost the expected style for use in business letters. But as time went on and more modern ideas came in, fashions in font style changed and more became available. Fonts tended to become simpler and some had no serifs, the small leg-like structures at the ends of characters (Figure 4.3).

While it was theoretically possible to take a typebar typewriter into a workshop and get the metal pieces that had the typeface on removed and new ones put in their place, this was rarely encountered and to all intents and purposes the typeface could be considered fixed.

The typewriter mechanism in most typebar typewriters was mechanical and manually operated (as opposed to electric devices). The depression of a key on the typewriter keyboard would require sufficient force to move a series of levers joined to the key and linked to the relevant typebar. If the key was hit fairly lightly, this would be translated into a fairly faint impact of the typebar onto the paper. A heavier depression of the key would create a greater impact on the paper. The typebars impacted onto the paper through a fabric typewriter ribbon that made the impacting typeface make an inked mark (the relevant typed character) on the page. The paper was held around a cylindrical

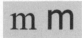

Figure 4.3 Letter **m** in a font with (left) and without (right) serifs.

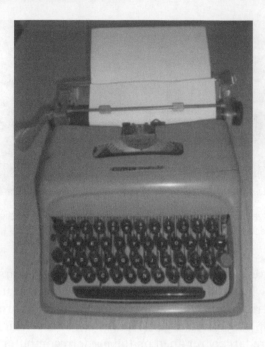

Figure 4.4   Paper inserted round a typewriter platen.

roller (or platen) (Figure 4.4). Rotation of the platen would move the paper
with it such that at the end of a line of typescript, the paper would wind around
the platen ready to start the next line a short distance below the previous line
(having essentially the same effect as pressing the ENTER key on a computer
keyboard). Most typewriters had a lever to set the distance between lines of
typescript at so-called single spacing, double or triple spacing (with a large
distance between lines of typing).

As each key stroke was made the platen (and hence the paper) would move
laterally a fixed distance. This ensured that each typed character had its own
place a fixed distance from the characters either side of it. This inter-letter
spacing was fixed for a given typebar typewriter, although different machines
could have different spacings, typically 10 characters per inch (often called
pica spacing) or 12 characters per inch (often called elite spacing).

The movement of the typebars themselves could vary depending on the
quality of the machine. The typebar was a moving and potentially slightly flexible arm bearing the typeface at its end. Any movement of the typebar (for
example from side to side) might alter the exact appearance and position of
the typed character on the paper. For example any twisting of the typebar
might cause the character to print unevenly (perhaps printing heavier at the
top of the letter for instance).

In general, large office machines were designed to withstand a lot of heavy
use and tended to be the most reliable in terms of the precision of the typescript produced using them. Smaller machines (often sold as portable devices

for home use) were sometimes less robust and there was a tendency for them to produce a somewhat more erratic and less precise typed product.

The fabric ribbons used in typebar typewriters were made from a woven material impregnated with ink. The ribbons were intended to be reused. New ribbons would produce a fairly well-inked, dark typed character, but with use, the amount of ink present in the ribbon would decrease and cause a correspondingly grey typed character. The weave pattern of the ribbon material and the diminution of ink present would tend to yield a typed character that became less clear in its appearance with a fuzzy outline (Figure 4.5).

In manual machines, the force with which a typewriter key is depressed is passed on to the typebar impacting onto the paper. (In electric typebar machines the keystroke led to an electrical signal going to the typebar and hence the force of the keystroke did not get translated into a heavier impact of the typebar onto the paper.) If the typed character was small, such as a fullstop, the force on that small character could punch through the paper surface, whereas the same force on a large character, such as a letter W, would be dispersed over a larger area and would not normally puncture the paper.

The evenness with which typewriter keys were depressed was to some extent related to training as a typist. Experienced typists had an even pressure that was generally reflected in the even ink deposition from the ribbon – the various typed characters were more or less of a similar ink colour intensity. In contrast, inexperienced typists were liable to depress typewriter keys with variable force leading to some characters being more intensely inked than others. This raised the possibility of being able to assess the quality not of the machine but of the operator, the typist. Skilled typing shares some similarity to handwriting in that it becomes a highly learned and automated skill with a variety of habits, such as the way that documents are formatted (Lines & Carodine, 2005).

The appearance of characters typed using a typebar typewriter can vary from one occasion to another depending on a number of factors. Obviously the typeface itself is constant, but the distribution of ink on a fabric ribbon

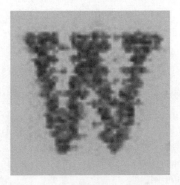

Figure 4.5 Close up of letter **w** showing the weave pattern from the fabric ribbon (x15 approx.).

may vary, the pressure with which the typeface comes into contact with the paper may vary depending on how hard the key is hit by the typist, and if the document is a carbon copy (used traditionally when typists wanted to produce multiple copies of a typed document – see Box 4.1) then it may be less well-defined in appearance.

Box 4.1 Carbon copy documents

Carbon paper consists of a thin flexible backing sheet coated on one side with a waxy ink-like material. A sandwich of sheets consisting of a top sheet of paper followed by a sheet of carbon paper (with the waxy side pointing away from the top sheet) and then a second sheet of paper would be inserted into the typewriter. The second sheet of paper would then take an imprint of the typescript via the ink on the carbon paper. The appearance of the carbon copy typescript was even fuzzier than that on the top copy through the fabric ribbon (Figure 4.6). The main reason for this was that the pressure of the typeface was reduced by the time it got through the top sheet and the carbon paper before reaching the second sheet of paper. Discerning the fine detail of the typeface, which as will be noted later is crucial in forensic examinations, was often very difficult when examining a carbon copy document. Indeed, it was not uncommon to use a second sheet of carbon paper and a third sheet of paper on to which a second copy of the typescript would be made, and the pressure on such a second copy would be even weaker and the detail of the typescript even less clear.

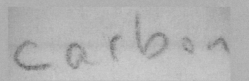

Figure 4.6 Close up of a carbon copy. *(See insert for colour representation of the figure.)*

An alternative to carbon paper was so-called No Carbon Required (NCR) documents. These were sets of pre-printed multiple-copy documents (such as invoices or order forms) where several (typically three or four) copies of a document were typed at the same time. The reverse of the NCR pages and the front of the page beneath were coated with materials which, when typed (or written) on caused chemicals from the two surfaces to mix and produce a visible dye.

If a small portable typewriter was used rather than a larger, heavy duty office machine this might lead to a more variable output from the less mechanically robust machine. So although there is no natural variation as there is in handwriting and signature production, there can still be variation in the both the clarity of the typed characters and their positioning on the line of typing from one occasion to another. This could affect the forensic examination if, for example, a letter **t** on some occasions appeared a fraction longer to the left and on others appeared a fraction longer to the right; in the absence of the typewriter itself, caution would be needed in interpreting this.

The typefaces used were sometimes supplied by separate manufacturers who would supply the same typeface to more than one typewriter manufacturer. As a consequence the same typeface could appear on typebar typewriters made by several different typewriter manufacturers. Over time a large number of typefaces became available for use on typebar typewriters. A number of typeface collections (see Box 4.2) were created with the purpose of enabling forensic document examiners to identify the make of machine used to type a document. In casework, requests for determining the manufacturer of a piece of typescript of unknown origin (so as to give investigators an idea of what to look for) were once common.

Box 4.2 Classifying typeface fonts

The first requirement is a collection of typefaces of known origin. These could be obtained from a variety of sources, such as a manufacturer's publicity material or typewriters examined in casework. The classification of typefaces in such a collection then requires a scheme that enables different typefaces to be distinguished. Since the different typefaces were based on fonts of different character shapes, the classification schemes would focus on certain letters, numerals or any other distinguishing features and define the form of the character into a number of categories. For example, the crossbar on the lower case letter **t** might be longer to the left or to the right of the upright. This one feature would not, of course, be enough to distinguish between the many hundreds of different typefaces, so for a system to work effectively typically 20–30 letters and numerals would be needed to adequately distinguish the many different typefaces. A small number of typescript classification schemes were created by a number of forensic investigation authorities around the world.

In general, classification schemes are best operated if a number of conditions are met. For a given feature (such as the letter **t** mentioned above) the distinctions between categories must be as clear as possible, bearing in mind that on a document typed using a fabric ribbon, the letter on the page may have a fuzzy, poorly defined appearance. As noted above, the appearance of a given character might vary slightly from one occasion to another and this may make it difficult to be sure which category is correct. For this reason, it is important that classification schemes can deal with uncertainty by not requiring all characters to be categorised and, if appropriate, using a Boolean approach (where a character is either Type 1 **or** Type 2 but **not** Type 3, for example).

Of course, for a classification scheme to work there must be a database of samples of known origin against which an unknown piece of typescript is compared. The production of a database must be done with great care since any errors that it contains may lead to not finding a match with a questioned sample of typescript. Two main types of error can occur. These are clerical (human) errors and classification errors in which a feature is incorrectly classified. Every effort needs to be made to minimise both kinds of error.

Searches based on classification schemes rarely yield unique results with just one matching hit in the database. If a piece of typescript has a number of its characters classified (such as the letters **a**, **f**, **g**, **I**, **m**, **t**, **E**, **M** and the numerals **4**, **7** and **8**) and the classifications are compared to a database, then it is often the case that a number of 'matches' will be found. In practice, therefore, it is often necessary and always wise to compare the questioned typescript with the actual typescript samples that were used to form the database, looking not just at the characters that went into the classification but also checking all of the other characters to make sure that they match too. It would not be beyond the realms of possibility in the example here that hits from the database differed in some *other* feature such as the letter **b** which had not formed part of the classification scheme.

The use of collections of typefaces was aimed almost exclusively at providing information to an investigator as to the make of machine involved in typing a document. Such databases had almost no value when comparing questioned and specimen typefaces, although they did have one useful function, namely to provide reference materials for examination. For example, if a questioned document showed a small letter **m** without a serif on its middle leg, should that be evidence that the serif was broken? Use of the reference collection of typefaces would show that some typefaces were *designed* with a letter **m** with no serif on its middle leg and hence the apparent broken serif might in fact be a design feature.

4.3   The forensic examination of typebar typewriters

Cases usually fall into one of two types. The first type requires a comparison between typed documents with samples produced on a particular typewriter with the machine being available for inspection. The second type of case is to show that a number of typed documents have (or have not) been typed on the same typewriter (there being no typewriter to examine).

When available, it is always good practice to examine a typewriter (or indeed any other device involved in forensic cases). The examination of a typewriter often follows a set routine. It is important to note the obvious features such as the make and model. The majority of typewriters are given serial numbers by their manufacturers which makes identifying the machine easier and can ensure that the machine examined in the laboratory by the document examiner is indeed the machine that ends up as a court exhibit some time later.

Most machines have a ribbon in place when submitted for forensic examination. The colour of the ribbon is generally just black but some typewriters were designed to be able to use two-colour ribbons, typically black at the top and red at the bottom with switching between colours made possible by moving a lever to slightly alter the position of the ribbon in the machine.

As noted above, the typescript produced by a typewriter may not always be crystal clear and there may be uncertainty about the fine detail that has been obscured by, for example, a fading ribbon. Direct examination of the typeface (on the ends of the typebars) using a hand lens will usually resolve any uncertainties.

Examination of the typeface can first and foremost determine whether or not it has been damaged. The typeface of a typebar typewriter is made of metal and it is therefore generally robust and not very likely to break. However, heavy use (exacerbated by heavy handed typing) can eventually lead to damage to the typeface. Such damage is very often focused on the weakest part of the characters, namely the serifs, the small leg-like elements present in many fonts (Figure 4.7). The nature of the metallic material is such that breaks tend to be sudden and complete – one day the serif is there, the next it has

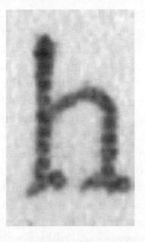

Figure 4.7 Close up of a letter **h** with top and bottom serifs on left side damaged (x15 approx.).

broken off; there is no gradual deterioration with first some loss of metal and then more over time. In fact the metal will have been cracking over a period of time but this will not be apparent from the typescript. Eventually the crack becomes such that the serif is no longer secure and it breaks away.

Damage of this kind is not uncommon, but on the other hand it is not by any means all that frequent. As far as the forensic document examiner is concerned, this is an ideal state of affairs since if no typeface ever deteriorated then that would make connecting typescripts to typewriters more difficult, and if such damage was too widespread many machines might show it and make it too commonplace to be significant. For the forensic document examiner, finding a damaged serif in some typescript is therefore of potentially considerable significance. Confirmation that the typeface has broken comes from an examination of the typeface on the typewriter that shows a break in the relevant part of the character where the serif used to be. Because the break is a fracturing process from the original smooth metal, the raw edge of the break appears uneven and under low power magnification this can be readily seen.

Damaged characters, then, provide the best evidence to link a typewriter to a document. But what if there are no damaged characters? As noted above, the positioning of typed characters on the page may be imperfect due to mechanical defects in such machines with typebars moving laterally or twisting, for example. The result is that typed characters may print to the left or right, above or below the line of typing or may ink more heavily in one part of the character than the other. Such misalignment defects are the next best source of evidence for the document examiner. Visualising misalignments can be done with the naked eye but it is helpful to use a grid of regular lines having the same inter-letter spacing as the typescript. Thus each character, if perfectly aligned, should fall into the centre of the grid boxes. However, the occurrence and variability of misalignments is often related to the type of typewriter, with more robust office machines generally showing fewer and less variable misalignments compared to smaller, portable machines that tend to show more misalignments of greater variability.

The next source of evidence is the cleanliness of the typeface. Paper fibres and typewriter ribbon ink often combine to produce a material that can accumulate into the typeface, especially filling in the closed loops of characters such as the letters **a**, **b d**, **e**, **g** and so on (Figure 4.8). Dirt accumulating in the typeface can be quite characteristic but it can also be transient, since it can either become so heavy that it drops out of its own accord or, if the typist is diligent, cleaned away using a small suitable brush.

Finally, the mechanism of the typewriter itself may become defective. Perhaps the most frequent example being the shift mechanism used to move between upper and lower case letters, for example. If this mechanism does not function properly, it can lead to all of the capital letters being out of alignment. An examination of the typewriter will often confirm the nature of the defect.

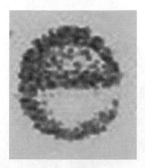

Figure 4.8 Close up of an infilled letter **e** (x15 approx.).

In some cases, however, a typewriter may not be available to examine. In such cases, the examination of the typed document is exactly the same but the option of confirming some details by examining the machine itself is not available. This can limit the interpretation of the observations made.

Interpreting evidence in cases involving typebar typewriters is based on the experience of the document examiner. As noted above, the most compelling evidence generally comes from damage defects, then misalignments, then dirt and mechanism defects. A number of considerations will show the basis for assessing the evidence. There are many typewriter manufacturers using different typefaces. If the typeface matches then that is already some evidence of a link between a document and either the typewriter or another document. But a match is, as noted above, a somewhat imprecise concept when there may be uncertainty about some tiny details of character shape obscured by a grey weave pattern from a ribbon. For this reason it may be better to use the notion of no discernible difference between the questioned and specimen typescripts in terms of the typeface. Likewise, the closeness of any similarity in damage defects, misalignments and dirt must also be treated with caution when there is uncertainty of detail. However, given, for example, some damaged characters and some marked and consistent misaligning of characters, it is possible to reach strong conclusions. If there are just one or two misalignments or slightly dirty characters then the evidence is weaker. Many document examiners use the same scale of opinion to express the strength of evidence in such cases as described for handwriting (see Section 2.9.2 in Chapter 2).

4.4 Single element typewriters

The reign of typebar typewriters in the office environment started to come to an end in the 1960s and was more or less over by the 1990s. The production of typewriters with removable typefaces was a major development during this change. Two types of machine were produced, one with the typeface on a sphere (so-called 'golfball' typewriters) and those with the typeface on a

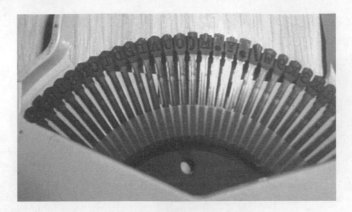

Figure 4.9   Showing a printwheel with one character at the end of each spoke (x2 approx.).

wheel (so-called printwheel or 'daisywheel' machines). The typing element (sphere or wheel) was made of plastic and contained the typeface either in a series of rows and columns on the sphere or at the end of spokes on the wheel (Figure 4.9).

These machines were devised so that the typeface could readily be changed by insertion of a new typing element. If the typeface became damaged, the old typing element could be discarded or if the typist wanted to change the appearance of the typescript, an element with a different typeface could be used. Such machines required electricity to work (to move the typing elements into the correct position). Depression of the typewriter keys would lead to rotation of the sphere in two dimensions (to bring the relevant row and column into place) prior to the sphere being impacted via a ribbon onto the paper. In machines using a wheel, key depression led to a spinning of the wheel until the relevant spoke was in place and a small hammer hit the back of the spoke to impact it through a ribbon onto the paper.

The mechanisms holding the typing elements in place and the movement of the elements during the typing process as each relevant character was brought into position for typing were generally more robust and precise in their operation as compared to typebar typewriters. As a result, the character alignment along the line of typing is generally good for single element machines, with fewer and less marked misalignments. Very small misalignments can be visualised by overlaying pieces of typescript with a view to highlighting any tiny discrepancies. Where single element typewriters lose forensic evidence in misalignments they more than make up for it in relation to damage defects. The golfball and daisywheel elements are made of plastic. This completely changes the nature of typeface damage compared to that seen with metal typebars. The nature of the plastic material is such that it will crack with wear and small pieces gradually break away. This gradual breakup of the plastic gives rise to very distinctive damage features (Figure 4.10).

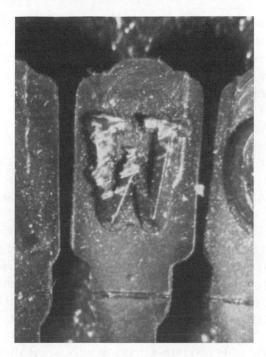

Figure 4.10 Close up of a severely damaged letter **w** on a printwheel (x10 approx.). *(See insert for colour representation of the figure.)*

It might be expected that the use of a particular letter would be related to the observed frequency of damaged letters. Letter usage in English begins with **e**, **t**, **a**, **o**, **i** and **n** as the most common and ends with **j**, **x**, **q** and **z** as the least common. However, a survey of typing elements showed that there was no relation between those characters showing damage and normal letter usage (Allen & Hardcastle, 1990). A possible explanation for this is that microscopic weaknesses were introduced into the plastic of the typing element during the manufacturing process. Only during typing did these weaknesses manifest themselves, starting with a tiny splitting of the plastic gradually becoming worse until a piece of plastic fell away from the typing element.

The conformation in which the golfball and daisywheel elements were made alters from one manufacturer to another so that typing elements from one machine may not fit into a similar kind of machine made by a different manufacturer. One consequence of this is that the range of different typefaces available for one machine can vary to those for a different machine. Also, the interchangeable nature of typing elements means that the damage defects are in fact on the typing element and not an integral part of the machine as a whole. Thus, the forensic link between a document and a single element type-writer is via the typing element. Since a typing element can be taken from one machine and put into another (compatible) machine, this has to be reflected in the way in which the evidence is reported so as to emphasise the link to the element and not the machine into which the element was fitted at a particular time (such as when seized by the authorities for forensic examination).

Single element machines also were designed to be used at more than one inter-letter spacing. For example, machines capable of typing at ten characters per inch and twelve characters per inch were available as traditionally found on many typebar typewriters. A new option was also possible on single element typewriters, namely proportional spacing. In proportional spacing the distance between characters along the line of typing depends on the width of the characters. A wide letter such as a **W** would be given more space to the next character than a narrow letter such as an **i**, thereby making the typescript appear more like the print in a book or magazine.

Yet another development during this period was machines that were capable of storing (small) amounts of text in a memory. For example, text could be typed in and the typewriter would store it temporarily until a full line of text was input and then the whole line would be typed out in one pass. The text could be viewed on a small display and this enabled the typist to check it prior to typing it on the page. These were primitive fore-runners of the word processing capability that was to become universal with the personal computer. The ability to store text rather than instantly type it after each key stroke led to the possibility of aligning the right hand margin of the typing (justified text), which was achieved by the typewriter inserting small spaces between words so as to leave the right hand margin aligned. Different typewriters do this using different means of calculating where the spaces are placed, and this provides another possible way of differentiating between typewriters.

4.5   Typewriter ribbons and correcting typescript

Typebar typewriters traditionally used ribbons made of ink-impregnated fabric which could be re-used. The appearance of the typing was darker with a new ribbon but faded with time as the ribbon was both re-used and the ink tended to dry.

As typewriters changed, so new ribbons were introduced. The most common was the plastic film ribbon, which was made from a narrow plastic tape with ink on one side, the ink being somewhat waxy in nature. Typing caused all of the ink from the relevant area of the ribbon to be transferred onto the paper, leaving an impression on the ribbon. The ink appeared very black and gave a clear edge to the typed character in contrast to the grey and uneven edges observed with fabric ribbons. As a consequence of all of the ink being transferred, such ribbons were intended to be used once only. Text typed using such a ribbon could readily be deciphered by reading the sequence of characters typed from the ribbon (Figure 4.11). Ribbons were used by different machines in different ways. All were held in a cassette, but some ribbons wound from left to right and some right to left, some had one, some had two and some three

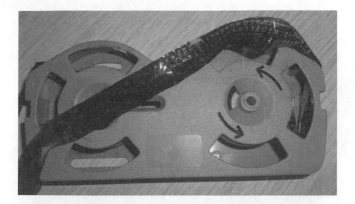

Figure 4.11 A carbon film ribbon showing readable text after use.

rows of text on wider ribbons with characters reading both from left to right (or vice versa) and top row to bottom row (or vice versa). Thus whilst deciphering the text was straightforward, it was made no easier by this additional complexity. Attempts were made to automate ribbon reading since manually transcribing a whole ribbon was very time consuming and if it was urgent then it could hold up an investigation. However, image processing in this period was fairly primitive and the devices produced to read ribbons essentially produced simply an image of the text on a sheet of paper (via a video camera and printer) making it easier to manipulate but still requiring human intervention to decipher and make sense of it.

4.5.1 Correcting typed documents

Documents produced using a fabric ribbon were difficult to correct because the ink impregnated the paper surface. Removal involved either physical abrasion of the paper using an eraser or covering up the error using an opaque (usually white) correcting fluid and typing over it, a process that often led to the transfer of residual correcting fluid onto the typeface, exacerbating the accumulation of dirt into the type face. Some machines were fitted with a correction ribbon that was coated on one side with correction fluid, the idea being that by going back to the error, the typist would use the correction ribbon to cover up the error and then (using the normal ribbon) type in the correct character. This method was not widely used.

The nature of the ink used with plastic film ribbons was such that it did not tend to impregnate the paper as much as ink from a fabric ribbon would. Rather the ink could be removed fairly easily from the surface of the paper leaving little disruption to the paper surface. This principle was used by fitting typewriters with a correction ribbon that again consisted of a plastic tape but with one side having a sticky surface which, when brought into contact with typescript, would lift the ink off the paper surface and transfer

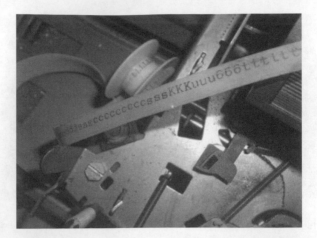

Figure 4.12　A lift off correction ribbon with removed characters present.

it to the sticky side of the tape. This process led to corrections lifted from a document in sequence also being readable by inspection of the correction ribbon (Figure 4.12). Despite removal of the ink, the indentation of the typed character into the paper surface remained.

In order to determine whether a document has been corrected using a correction ribbon, the paper surface has to be examined carefully using an oblique light source to locate any impression into the paper surface. If, for example, several words have been corrected off the page, they will appear on the correction ribbon and also leave indentations on the page (although if new text were typed over the lifted off characters this could obscure the indentations to some extent). In principle, a sequence of characters removed from a page as shown by the remaining indentations can be linked forensically to a corresponding sequence of characters appearing on the correction ribbon of a typewriter.

Box 4.3　Dating typed documents

In some cases the date on which a document was typed is the key question being asked of the document examiner.

One possibility is that the typeface used was not available on the date shown by the document. If it is possible to determine, for example using a database of typefaces, which typeface was used and to contact relevant manufacturers to gain background information as to when it was first used, it might be possible to show that the typeface was not available at the date in question.

A second approach would be to examine a chronological sequence of documents known to have been typed using the machine in question. If those documents revealed a gradual deterioration of the typescript in terms of damage, misalignments or even dirt in the typeface, then the questioned document can be compared to that sequence to see where best it fits and hence estimate a date of production. With plastic typing elements the scope for such a chronology is particularly good due to the gradual deterioration of damaged characters over time, and this was exactly the method of examination used by Hardcastle (1986) who observed gradual break up of a letter **k** and was able to show that a document in question was not produced on the date shown on the document.

4.6 Computer printers

Over a period of years, the typewriter as a standalone device became less and less used and the printer as an add-on to computers took over. During this transition period, a number of devices appeared and soon disappeared. Three have dominated the printer market. Initially, impact matrix printers were very widely used then, as technology and market forces developed, laser and inkjet became dominant.

4.6.1 Impact matrix printers

Computer printers generally create text and images from a pattern of dots or matrix. With impact matrix printers, the dots were created by impacting pins through a ribbon onto the paper. Because of the impact and the small cross-section of the pin head, the ribbons needed to be robust and fabric ribbons were generally used. A character of text was made up of a pattern of pin impressions. The pins were arranged in one or two rows in a vertical line in the print head, which moved from side to side across the paper. Typically there were nine pins in a row with seven above the print line and two below for the tails of letters such as **g** and **y**. The pins were fired in the correct pattern in order to make up recognisable letters and numerals (Figure 4.13). The order in which the pins were fired was determined by software.

At the time of manufacture, the pins were equally spaced from one another and fell in a perfect vertical line. However, with use the pins could become bent and produce dots either displaced to the side, or too close to the pin above or below, effectively forms of misalignment defect that could provide a forensic link either between documents or with a particular printer and its print head.

For a time, impact matrix printers tried to move into the image printing market by using coloured ribbons, with a picture being made up of a series of passes using different colours on a ribbon. This was an extremely slow process and produced images of generally poor quality, and laser and inkjet soon took

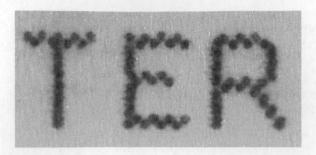

Figure 4.13   Matrix characters are made up of a pattern of dots (x15 approx.).

over. One advantage that impact matrix printers had over laser and inkjet was that the latter two are non-impact technologies. Where it was efficient to type onto multiple copy documents such as invoice sets, this could be done with impact matrix printers but not laser or inkjet.

4.6.2   Laser printers

Laser printers use toner technology similar to that used in photocopiers. The text or image is digital (determined by computer software) and it causes a laser beam to move across a light-sensitive metal cylindrical drum. The effect of the light on the drum is to change its electrostatic properties in the area concerned. This electrostatic charge can attract toner material which can then be transferred to a sheet of paper. The toner is fused to the paper using heat and pressure. The cylindrical drum is then cleaned of residual toner and is available for the next laser illumination.

Toner is a chemically complex material that has a granular appearance when viewed under low power microscopy (Figure 4.14). The toner is a solid material that tends not to diffuse very much into the paper surface but rather sits on it. The deposition of toner onto the paper is mostly in the image area (be it text or pictures), but there is usually a background scatter of individual toner particles across the paper surface too.

The cylindrical drum can, with use, develop small imperfections on its surface. These imperfections may attract toner particles such that each time documents are printed using it there will be a characteristic mark on the paper. The position and shape of such marks can provide forensic evidence linking documents printed using the same laser printer (specifically the drum) or linking documents to a particular printer. The drum marks are often very small and require low power magnification to be seen.

Given the likelihood of a background scatter of toner particles on a document, it is important to distinguish them from marks caused by drum defects. A difference between them is that background scatter is random whereas drum marks will appear repeatedly on documents, usually in the same relative position one to another on the document. The diameter of

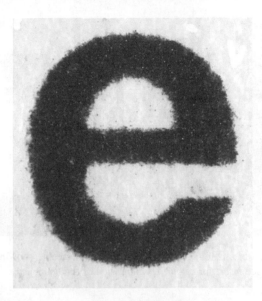

Figure 4.14 Letter **e** printed with a laser printer showing the molten appearance of raised toner on a paper surface (x30 approx.). *(See insert for colour representation of the figure.)*

many laser printer drums is quite small such that to print a sheet of A4 paper requires perhaps three rotations of the drum. This will cause the drum mark to appear three times down the page spaced equally apart. Background scatter usually consists of one or a few toner particles, whereas drum marks often have a shape associated with them (Figure 4.15). Any shape to drum marks will add to their forensic significance.

The use of colour in laser printers is made possible by having (usually) four toners available in yellow, cyan, magenta and black. These colours can be

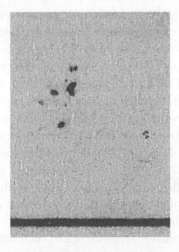

Figure 4.15 Close up of a group of drum defects (x15 approx.).

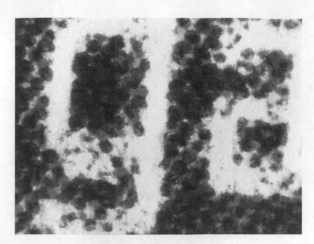

Figure 4.16   Close up of a colour laser print showing four colour (showing as shades of grey) dots (x30 approx.). *(See insert for colour representation of the figure.)*

combined to produce many different colours. Each colour is printed onto the paper separately and in sequence. What might appear to be a solid colour to the naked eye will be shown to be made up of a combination of these colours when viewed under the microscope (Figure 4.16).

The chemical composition of the toner material can be analysed using a variety of techniques (see Section 4.8.3 below and also Chapter 7 for further discussion of the techniques used).

4.6.3   The forensic examination of laser printers and laser printed documents

The first step when examining a document is to establish whether it has been produced on a laser printer. This involves low power microscopy to confirm the presence of toner material. Next the document needs to be viewed under magnification for any potential drum marks. Since these can be tiny and not always easy to differentiate from background scatter, the identity of a drum mark may be confirmed by finding it repeated along the sheet of paper or by finding a mark in the same place on several pages of laser printed documents.

If a laser printer is available for examination it will be necessary to take some specimen sheets from it in order to compare any drum marks that it shows with those on the documents of interest. If drum marks are found, their forensic significance will depend on the number of marks and their distinctiveness (in particular, their shape). It is a matter of the expert's judgement as to the strength of evidence, but if there are sufficient distinctive marks then a very strong evidential link may be justified.

A number of factors must be considered in such cases, however (which will also be relevant when considering photocopy documents). In general, defects to any object are non-reversible unless there is some sort of intervention (such as the servicing of a machine). It is also likely that either some defects will become worse over time or that new defects will appear (or both). This will require careful interpretation when comparing defect marks on documents that were perhaps allegedly produced on a machine some months before the specimens were taken from it at the time of the examination. Given the tendency for defects to worsen and accumulate, there may be an apparent mismatch between the older documents and the newer (and hence potentially more defective) specimens. The reasoning process that needs to be used is this: Could the defect pattern shown by the older document be a forerunner of that seen in the contemporary specimen? If so, how much evidence (in terms of the number and distinctiveness of any defects) is there to support that possibility?

4.6.4 Inkjet printers

Inkjet printers build text and images from a large number of drops of ink. The ink used is a liquid ink that tends to soak into the paper's surface (Figure 4.17), in marked contrast to the solid toner that is used in laser printers that sits on the surface of the paper. This type of printer has become more and more commonplace as its cost has fallen and technology has improved, for example reducing drop size down to the level of picolitres (10^{-12} litre). The smaller the drop size, the better the quality of the image produced.

There are two main kinds of inkjet printer that are differentiated by the method of delivering the ink to the page. Drop-on-demand printers will only produce a drop of ink when it is needed by the printer (as directed by software). Continuous ink printers send out a stream of droplets from the

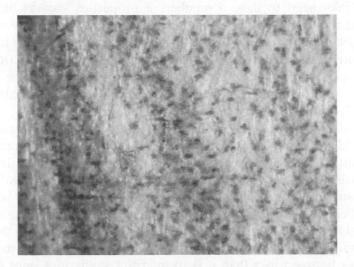

Figure 4.17 Close up of inkjet printing with ink absorbed into paper (x30 approx.). *(See insert for colour representation of the figure.)*

print head. When a drop is required at a particular location it is allowed to hit the paper, but when it is not required, the ink is deflected back into the ink reservoir to be recycled. The process of ejecting ink from the print head varies between machines but can include heat or piezoelectric crystals (which change their dimensions when charged with electricity and thus can expel ink from the print head). Print heads therefore contain both the mechanism for ejecting ink from the tiny pinhole openings in them and also reservoirs of ink.

As with laser printers, inkjet printers typically have four inks available (cyan, magenta, yellow and black) from which a vast array of colours can be made by using different combinations. What appear to be solid colours to the naked eye will be shown to be made up of dots of ink under magnification.

Inkjet drops that are ejected from the print head are usually accompanied by a halo of tiny micro-droplets (often called satellites), which also soak into the paper and create a fine haze around the main printed image/text. Because of the lateral movement of the print head across the page as it releases its ink droplets, the fine haze tends to be more apparent behind the direction of movement and hence under microscopic examination it is possible to determine the direction of travel of the print head across the page.

4.6.5　The forensic examination of inkjet printers

The appearance of the ink under low power magnification may show slightly differing colours of ink, different drop sizes and arrangements and possibly different degrees of satellite droplet formation. If microscopy is unable to distinguish between different inkjet-printed documents, chemical analysis may be appropriate.

The composition of inks used in inkjet printers varies between suppliers. The inks need to have a number of properties such as being fluid, remaining colour-fast on the paper and able to resist various environmental factors such as bright light and oxidation. The chemical analysis of inkjet inks can be carried out using a number of techniques, including electrophoresis (for example, Szafarska et al., (2011)), Raman spectroscopy (for example, Heudt et al., (2012)) and mass spectrometry (Houlgrave et al., (2013)). (See Chapter 7 for further discussion of these techniques.)

If it is not possible by the means available to distinguish between inkjet inks, the identification of a particular inkjet printer (or, more precisely its print head) as having produced a particular document is extremely difficult. Occasionally there may be disruption to the electronic signals to the print head causing a failure of ink release leading to, for example, a whole row of dots being missing on the printout. Such failures may provide some additional evidence to link documents either to each other or to the printer itself if available. As with many forensic investigations, it is easier to interpret differences between inks than it is to interpret similarities since the latter requires information relating to how common the particular inks are.

For the vast majority of cases, inkjet inks will be those widely available in retail outlets. However, it is possible for bespoke inkjet inks to be produced, for example to produce letterheads in house. Microscopic examination would still show the characteristic appearance of inkjet inks, but there might be only one colour present rather than the colour being a composite made up of cyan, yellow, magenta and black. By their very nature, such inks are far less frequently encountered and their presence may be of forensic significance.

Box 4.4 Dye sublimation printing

Laser and inkjet printed documents dominate the market at present and, in casework terms, are by far the most likely to be encountered. However, there are other printer technologies such as dye sublimation.

In dye sublimation printing, the solid ink is held on a substrate from which it is rapidly heated to a gaseous state with no intermediate liquid phase (the process known as sublimation). The ink interacts with the paper and forms the image. Such inks may also be used on other media such as plastic. The ink has a waxy appearance and has a stepped form under low power magnification caused by the heating process.

4.7 Fax (facsimile) machines

Fax machines were originally developed to send text and images along telephone lines. In order to achieve this, the text and images had to be digitised and the digitised information could then be sent along the telephone line where, at the receiving end, the information was decoded to reconstruct the text and image for printing out. This was originally a fairly crude process due to limitations in the technology, and as a result the document that was received and printed out had poor resolution and a block-like appearance. Each small block of the printed fax copy document corresponded to the area of the original document, which was either coded as black or white with no intermediate grey tones. If there was more black than white in a block area it was coded as black and vice versa.

The printing process at the receiving fax machine was usually thermal, with the printer often set up with heat-sensitive paper. Each time there was a 'black' block to print, an electrode in the printer mechanism would heat up causing the paper in that small area to darken. Each time there was a white block then the mechanism would pass on leaving the paper still white. The crude nature of the 'copying' process and the mechanical process of paper moving through the printer led to frequent distortion of the printout in comparison to the original, including small dimensional changes.

Determining whether or not a given fax-printed document could have been printed on a particular fax machine may involve not only the examination of the printer but also the capability of the sending machine. This is particularly the case when the header or footer details that typically appeared on fax documents are relevant, since they are determined by the sending machine.

4.8 Photocopiers

The examination of photocopy documents can occur in a number of contexts. In the world of business, it is common for documents to be copied (first generation copy) and copied again (second generation copy) and so on. Forensic document examiners often examine aspects of a document from a copy. For example, handwriting or a signature may have to be examined from a copy document when the original is no longer available.

However, some cases involve the examination of photocopy documents in order to determine, for example, the photocopier on which it was produced. These cases are often very difficult because of the simple way in which a copy can be first, second or whatever generation, a process that introduces many potential pitfalls.

Photocopy technology today has become somewhat standardised, with machines using a solid toner-based system of creating the image or text on the paper. Solid toner has a characteristic appearance when viewed under a low power microscope – see Figure 4.14. In the past, some machines used a liquid toner, but such machines are almost never encountered any more.

The process of getting the toner onto the paper is essentially the same as for a laser printer described in Sections 4.6.2 and 4.6.3. The purpose of a photocopier was to simply reproduce in copy form a pre-existing image or text. By placing it onto a glass surface (usually called the platen) and using an optical mechanism, the details to be copied switch on or off a light source that is aimed at a light-sensitive metal drum inside the copier – as in a laser printer. In the past, this process was an analogue process involving mirrors and lenses. Modern photocopiers use digital scanning technology and this gives the potential to then manipulate the image using computer software prior to any print out of the copied details. In addition, the use of colour copiers has increased as the cost of the machines has fallen. Most colour copiers use four separate colours to generate the many different colours that can be achieved by mixing different proportions of cyan, magenta and yellow together with black. Different microscopic amounts of each colour are deposited on the paper in such a way that the human eye perceives the printed product as solid colour. It is only by using magnification that it becomes apparent that the print is composed of many small deposits of coloured toner particles.

Since photocopiers and laser printers use the same basic technology, the printed product when viewed under the microscope is the same. And since laser printers linked to a computer and scanner are to all intents and purposes using the same technology as inside a photocopier, then it is simplest to say that a document has been produced using toner rather than try and determine the exact type of machine used.

Photocopy documents are probably more likely to be copies of copies than laser printed documents if only for the reason that a laser printed document is often held as a computer file whereas an existing copy of a document is most conveniently copied again on a photocopier (thereby avoiding the need to scan and file on a computer). As a practical process, photocopying is quicker and more convenient.

4.8.1 The forensic examination of copy documents

There are a number of lines of examination that can be followed. Each case must be assessed on its own merits as to which approach is best.

The glass platen can be marked. Some marks may be transitory, such as a hair or some extraneous correction fluid. Glass is difficult to scratch but if it is scratched then this may provide a unique mark that becomes visible on the copy document.

Another important source of evidence comes from defects that accumulate on the light sensitive drum, which may become scratched and then such scratches will appear on the paper surface as small extraneous areas of toner. The shape and position of the marks will be highly characteristic as they are random in their occurrence.

The position of defect marks on the copy document may indicate whether the defect is caused by an imperfection on the platen or on the drum. The circumference of the light sensitive drum will affect how many turns it makes to produce a copy (which is also influenced by the size of the copy, be it A4 or A3, for example). The number of rotations of the drum to produce the standard A4 copy may vary from less than one (if the drum has a large circumference) to about three rotations (if the drum has a small circumference). Hence, a mark that repeats a couple of times down the page is strongly indicative of a drum defect. Also, if the defect is large and appears to have been caused by a hair, for example, this is probably a platen defect. However, a defect mark may not be visible if it happens to coincide with the printed details on a particular copy document. This might be a particular problem where the document has a lot of image and text and little unprinted (white paper) areas, such as banknotes.

If two copy documents share the same set of defect marks, then there is a temptation to assume that both documents were produced on the same photocopier. However, as noted above, it is easy for a copy of a copy to be made, and so the document examiner needs to consider the possibility, for example where two documents share some defect marks, that one copy document was created on a first photocopier and that this copy was subsequently copied on a second copier to produce the other copy document.

There are many routes to producing copy documents and it is often not possible to be absolutely certain of what has happened. In order to deal with this complex situation, there are a few 'rules' that can be used.

The first rule is that a copy document cannot be as clear as the document from which it is copied since the copying process is imperfect. Or put another way, it is impossible to create a clear copy from an unclear original document.

Another point to consider is that photocopiers usually can have the amount of toner reduced by lowering the contrast setting on the machine. The lowering of the contrast might produce a fainter copy such that some small or faint details that are present on the original do not show up on the copy.

Photocopiers do not always make exact 1:1 dimension copies. A dimension distortion of 1 or 2% is not unusual and this may be both down and across the sheet or just in one direction.

The changes in detail shown and dimensional distortions shown by copy documents may assist the expert in determining the relationship between various copies derived from the same original document. Of course, handwritten text is essentially unique and when copied there can be no question that ultimately there was only one original piece of handwriting. In contrast, modern computer-printed text can be printed from a saved computer file time and again, each printout being essentially identical to another, albeit the position of the text on the page or the type of printer used may vary.

4.8.2   Composite documents

Based on the many ways in which copy documents can be manipulated, it is possible to create a bogus document from genuine original components. Text, both printed and handwritten, and images can be copied either using a photocopier or by scanning into a computer. Manipulation of the information by cutting, pasting, cropping and the addition of new text or images can then produce a completely fraudulent document. Using the examination methods described above, the expert may be able to determine how the bogus document was produced or, failing that, it may be possible to suggest a number of ways it might have been produced.

4.8.3   Analysis of toner

Apart from an examination of the image content of a copy document, be it text or pictures or handwriting, the physical material from which it is composed, the toner, can be analysed. The toner typically contains colorant (dyes or pigments), a binder and other additives to ensure that it has the required chemical and physical properties.

Over the years in which photocopy technology has developed, a large number of analytical procedures to discriminate between different toners have been used (see Chapter 7). Amongst these are methods that fall into the categories of infrared spectroscopy (for example, Kemp and Totty, (1983)), x-ray fluorescence (for example, Trzcinska, (2006)), gas chromatography (for example, Egan et al., (2003)) and Raman spectroscopy (for example, Bozicevic et al., (2012)). However, there are a number of variants of these techniques and other analytical techniques that have also been used.

Analysis of toner clearly requires the availability of the necessary chemical equipment and the expertise to interpret the findings. In many cases a visual examination will be sufficient but chemical analysis may be a fruitful next approach if a visual examination does not assist the investigation.

From the descriptions in this chapter of methods for examining typed and copied documents, it is clear that some methods do not involve damaging the document, such as low power microscopy. However, chemical analysis can require removal of material from the document and these so-called destructive techniques, while usually only requiring tiny samples of material, nonetheless are altering the document. For this reason it is important that no destructive examinations are carried out without permission from an appropriate authority, such as the investigator. In addition, it is important to make a record (for example, a good quality photograph) of what the document looks like before any material is removed for analysis. The place(s) from which any material is removed should be recorded as this should then correspond to any (minor) areas of disruption to the document's surface that will be apparent afterwards.

In general, non-destructive techniques are quicker and cheaper than destructive techniques and often provide the evidence needed. However, analytical methods may be justified where no other evidence has been adduced.

4.9 Case notes in cases involving typed and copied documents

The amount of detail that needs to go into notes in cases involving typed or printed documents will vary from one case to another. In typescript cases involving traditional typewriters, it would be wise to place on file a photocopy of some documents as a record of the typeface. If there are any defects of the typescript, such as broken or misaligned characters, these can be highlighted on the file copy or sketched in the notes or both to indicate not just the presence of a defect but also its nature, be it a broken or a misaligned character. Inter-letter spacing should be noted for documents typed on typewriters. Any alterations to the typescript should be noted and the method of altering recorded (such as use of a correction ribbon) and any text that has been removed but that can be deciphered from its impression on the paper surface should be noted since it may be possible to link this to text found on a correction ribbon at a later date.

If a typewriter or printer is available for examination, then any model and serial numbers must be recorded so that at a later time it is possible to be sure about which machine was examined. Any specimens taken from typewriters or printers should be clearly labelled and retained on the file. If a typewriter ribbon is removed for deciphering, it is usually necessary to break into the cassette in which it is held – this process must be recorded appropriately.

With photocopy documents, it is a good idea to compare defect marks and their placement by using a clear plastic sheet and marking on it, using a suitable pen, where the marks are and, where appropriate, their shape. This transparency can then be overlaid on other documents to determine which defect marks correspond and which do not. If a copier itself is available, again any model and serial numbers should be noted. Obtaining specimens might require the placing of a blank sheet of paper on the platen and obtaining a series of perhaps 6–12 photocopies from the machine. The sequence with which they emerge from the machine should be recorded in case there are any unexpected changes in defect mark pattern with use.

If a questioned document is a photocopy and this is then photocopied by the expert to form part of the case record, it is crucial that the copies do not get muddled up. To minimise this risk, any copy document produced by the expert should be immediately marked as a file copy and the questioned document returned to a safe place where its identity is known (such as any packaging in which it was submitted).

Whatever the means of production of a typed or printed document, the observations that lead to the identification of the process must be recorded, which almost always will require a description of findings using microscopy. In addition, some print processes may be identified in part by features that they *do not* exhibit and so negative findings can also usefully be noted. For example, the absence of toner particles would rule out laser and photocopy processes or the absence of impressions in the paper surface will probably rule out conventional typewriters.

Having recorded relevant observations, it is important to consider what possible explanations there may be for them in the context of the particular case. In photocopy cases in particular this can be very difficult because of the possibility of making copies of copies. Likewise, documents produced on computer printers may be derived from a saved word processing file capable of being printed off on more than one occasion. As a result, the expert may only be able to come to fairly general conclusions as to how a document came into being. In such cases, it might be instructive to consider the evidence of witnesses who claim to know how the documents were produced because it is sometimes possible to refute such evidence. Even if positive evidence is not feasible it may be possible to say how a document *was not* produced even if it is not possible to be sure how it *was* produced.

Many other features of the documents may need to be recorded depending on the documents concerned, how they have been produced and what allegations may have been made regarding their production – for example that a document is bogus and is a composite made up from parts of other documents. The notes must be a record from which the process of examination is clear and which provide the key findings that form the basis of any conclusions to which the expert comes. The significance of findings may need to be assessed both individually and collectively so that there is transparent justification for the opinions expressed.

4.10 Reports in cases involving typed and copied documents

Typewriters, computer printers and copiers of various kinds are pieces of machinery that are, to varying degrees, familiar to large sections of the public in general and professional people in particular as they are tools of the trade for many people. That does not mean that they have a good knowledge or understanding of how the devices work and still less about how the forensic expert examines them and documents are produced on them. However, it does mean that some aspects of these machines' function can be regarded as general knowledge – such as what a photocopier or computer printer does, even if how it does it is not so widely known. The expert's report in cases involving these devices can therefore build upon this basic general understanding by linking it to more technical details. For example, the notion of letter design in typewriters or the possibility of extraneous marks on photocopies can be described in ways that are readily understood by the non-expert.

The report must contain enough information to enable the reader to follow the path from the question (such as 'was the questioned document copied on this copier?') to the conclusion reached by the expert. The key findings (such as defect marks) that justify the conclusion must be described using non-technical language as far as possible. With any case involving these devices, the alternative explanation centres on the notion that another device (of the same model and manufacturer, for example) could have been used instead and this issue must therefore be considered explicitly in the report.

In addition, in cases involving copy documents, there may be many possible paths (copies of copies) by which the questioned document could have been created, and it is often difficult to concisely describe these and indeed impossible to exhaustively consider *all conceivable* paths. To ensure that the report remains comprehensible to the reader, it is a good idea to enumerate some possible pathways and to indicate how the evidence available either supports or refutes the likelihood of the various options.

Because reports in these cases can become involved and intricate, it is especially important that there is a summary that describes the final conclusion without the explanatory reasoning so that the reader is left in no doubt as to what the expert is saying and can seek the reasoning elsewhere in the report.

Typescript comparison: a worked example

In this section an example of how to approach a case and make notes is demonstrated. It should be stressed that there are a number of different ways to make notes and the intention here is to show the kinds of issues that need to be considered and how these interrelate with the observation process leading to a conclusion.

Case circumstances

Mr Jackson and Mr Doyle have been having disputes about property boundaries for a number of years. Two anonymous letters have been received by Mr Jackson who says that Mr Doyle sent them to him and is claiming harassment.

Purpose

To compare the typescripts on items 1 and 2 to determine if they have been typed on the same typewriter.

Items submitted

Item 1: Note – Dear Mr Jackson (Figure 4.18)

Item 2: Note – Like father like son (Figure 4.19)

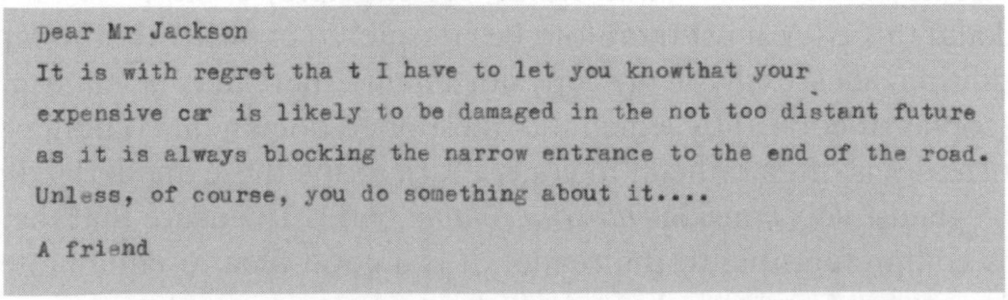

```
Dear Mr Jackson
It is with regret tha t I have to let you knowthat your
expensive car is likely to be damaged in the not too distant future
as it is always blocking the narrow entrance to the end of the road.
Unless, of course, you do something about it....

A friend
```

Figure 4.18   Worked example: Note item 1.

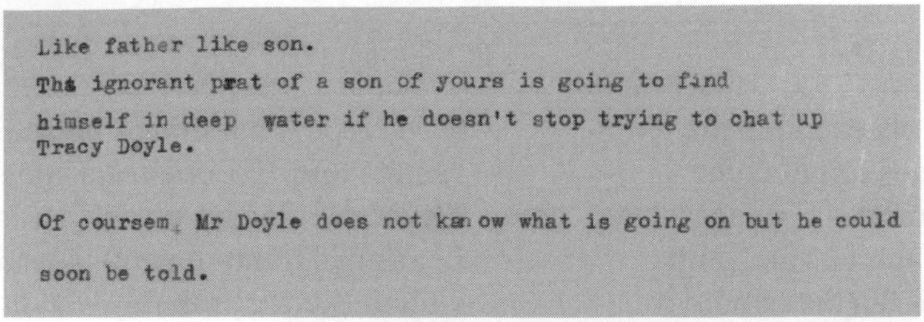

```
Like father like son.
The ignorant prat of a son of yours is going to find
himself in deep  water if he doesn't stop trying to chat up
Tracy Doyle.

Of coursem  Mr Doyle does not kan ow what is going on but he could

soon be told.
```

Figure 4.19   Worked example: Note item 2.

Case notes

Observations	Thoughts
• Close inspection shows the weave pattern typical of a fabric ribbon. • The typed characters are indented into the paper surface.	Examination of the two notes to see if they are original typescript or copies of some kind. This shows that the typescript is original and not a copy.
Fabric ribbon often associated with typebar machines but could be used by other types of machine. • Poor alignment of typed characters noted such as **D** of Dear and **ar** in car in item 1 and. • **D** in Doyle and **t** in what in item 2. Inking is very variable with some characters being more heavily inked than others suggesting manual machine (possibly with an unskilled operator).	What sort of typewriter was used'? Poor alignment and uneven inking typical of typebar machines and would be most unusual in single element machines.

Observations	Thoughts
Carefully examine the letter shapes for all typed characters. All characters are similar between the two items.	Are the type fonts similar between items 1 and 2? Look for any clear differences in any single character bearing in mind the grey fabric ribbon (hence probably well used) leads to poor clarity and definition of character shape.
Measure the spacing between letters and compare the size of typed characters to see if they are the same: they are similar.	Is the inter-letter spacing and size of the typed characters similar between items 1 and 2?

Up to this point all observations are consistent with the two documents having been typed on the same typewriter. However, more evidence is needed before coming to a firm conclusion since it is possible that they were typed on two different typewriters that coincidentally have the same typeface.

It is very difficult to determine how common or rare a particular typeface is, especially now since typewriters are not so frequently encountered.

Noted that: • some capital letters print low on both items, • letter **o** prints high, • letter **t** prints to right, • some letters showing infill from dirt such as letters **o**, **e**, **a** and **h**. • No damage defects noted although difficult to be certain because of poor definition of typed characters with a well-used ribbon. All characters must be compared to show all such defects of the typescript.	In order to get some stronger evidence, look for defects of the typescript that are similar or different between items 1 and 2. These can be damage defects, misalignments or dirt accumulation.

Summary
- Type fonts are similar shape and size and spacing.
- Further evidence from similar poor alignment and infilling of some characters, but no clear-cut damage to typeface.

Alternative explanations:

1. The two items were typed on the same typewriter.
2. The two items were typed on different typewriters.

Conclude that there is some strong evidence that items 1 and 2 were typed on the same typewriter but in the absence of damage to the typeface and more characteristic misalignments, the possibility of two different typewriters having been used cannot be completely ruled out although the evidence makes that possibility unlikely.

Report of Forensic Expert

Qualifications and experience ...

Scope of expertise ...

Items examined

I have examined the following items at the instruction of (the investigating authority). They were received at the laboratory on (dates).

Item 1: Note – Dear Mr Jackson

Item 2: Note – Like father like son

Purpose

I have compared the typescripts on items 1 and 2 with a view to determining whether or not they were typed on the same typewriter.

Findings

The typescripts on items 1 and 2 are similar in spacing and letter design one to the other. They also show a number of significant similarities in misalignment and dirt infilling to the typeface, although no damage is apparent to the typeface. The typescript on both items is typical of that produced on a traditional typebar typewriter.

In my opinion, there is strong evidence that items 1 and 2 were typed on the same typewriter but the possibility that two different machines were used cannot be completely ruled out, although I consider this possibility to be unlikely.

Summary

There is strong evidence that the two notes, items 1 and 2, were typed using the same typewriter.

References

Allen, M. J., & Hardcastle, R. A. (1990). The distribution of damage defects among characters of printwheel typing elements. *Forensic Science International*, 47(3), 249–259.

Bozicevic, M. S., Gajovic, A., & Zjakic, I. (2012). Identifying a common origin of toner printed counterfeit banknotes by micro-raman spectroscopy. *Forensic Science International*, 223(1–3), 314–320. doi:10.1016/j.forsciint.2012.10.007.

Egan, W. J., Galipo, R. C., Kochanowski, B. K., et al. (2003). Forensic discrimination of photocopy and printer toners. III. Multivariate statistics applied to scanning electron microscopy and pyrolysis gas chromatography/mass spectrometry. *Analytical and Bioanalytical Chemistry*, 376(8), 1286–1297. doi:10.1007/s00216-003-2099-3.

Hardcastle, R. A. (1986). Progressive damage to plastic printwheel typing elements. *Forensic Science International*, 30(4), 267–274.

Heudt, L., Debois, D., Zimmerman, T. A., et al. (2012). Raman spectroscopy and laser desorption mass spectrometry for minimal destructive forensic analysis of black and color inkjet printed documents. *Forensic Science International*, 219(1–3), 64–75. doi:10.1016/j.forsciint.2011.12.001.

Houlgrave, S., LaPorte, G. M., Stephens, J. C., & Wilson, J. L. (2013). The classification of inkjet inks using AccuTOF DART (direct analysis in real time) mass spectrometry. A preliminary study. *Journal of Forensic Sciences*, 58(3), 813–821. doi:10.1111/1556-4029.12048.

Kemp, G. S., & Totty, R. N. (1983). The differentiation of toners used in photocopy processes by infrared-spectroscopy. *Forensic Science International*, 22(1), 75–83. doi:10.1016/0379-0738(83)90121-4.

Lines, S. R., & Carodine, R. B. (2005). A study of business letter features. *Journal of Forensic Sciences*, 50(4), 924–927.

Szafarska, M., Wietecha-Posluszny, R., Wozniakiewicz, M., & Koscielniak, P. (2011). Application of capillary electrophoresis to examination of color inkjet printing inks for forensic purposes. *Forensic Science International*, 212(1–3), 78–85. doi:10.1016/j.forsciint.2011.05.017.

Trzcinska, B. M. (2006). Classification of black powder toners on the basis of integrated analytical information provided by fourier transform infrared spectrometry and X-ray fluorescence spectrometry. *Journal of Forensic Sciences*, 51(4), 919–924. doi:10.1111/j.1556-4029.2006.00167.x.

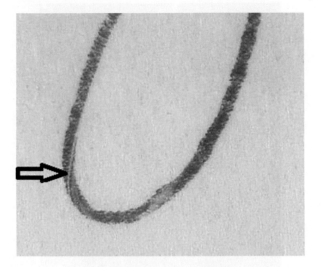

Figure 2.6   Striation lines in a ballpoint pen ink line (×10 approx.).

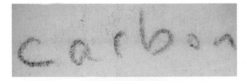

Figure 4.6   Close up of a carbon copy.

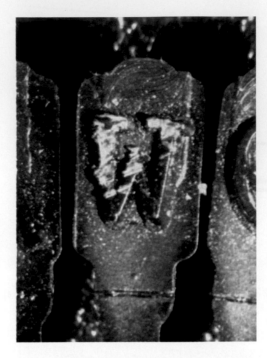

Figure 4.10 Close up of a severely damaged letter **w** on a printwheel (×10 approx.).

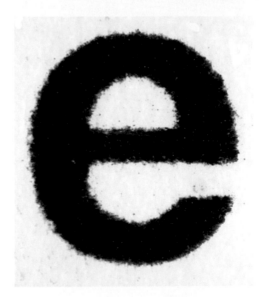

Figure 4.14 Letter **e** printed with a laser printer showing the molten appearance of raised toner on a paper surface (×30 approx.).

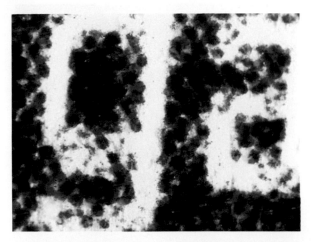

Figure 4.16 Close up of a colour laser print showing four colour (showing as shades of grey) dots (×30 approx.).

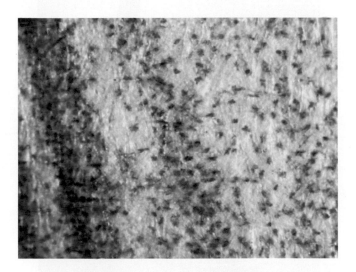

Figure 4.17 Close up of inkjet printing with ink absorbed into paper (×30 approx.).

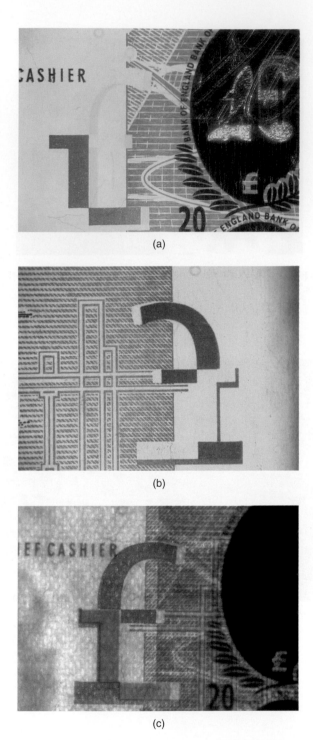

Figure 5.1 (a) The symbol on the front of the currency note; (b) the symbol on the reverse of the currency note; (c) the currency note viewed with transmitted light giving the completed symbol (×4 approx.).

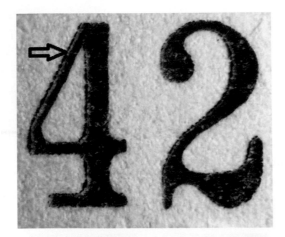

Figure 5.4 Ink squash around the edge of printed characters (×25 approx.).

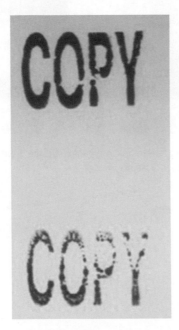

Figure 5.5 Stamp impressions vary in appearance depending on different conditions of applying. The upper stamp impression has been applied more heavily than the lower impression.

Figure 5.6 The gradual merging of colours found in split duct printing.

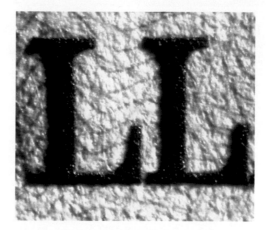

Figure 5.7 Close up showing raised ink on paper surface from a recessed printing process viewed under oblique lighting (×25 approx.).

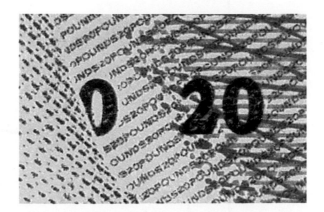

Figure 5.8 Microprinting (×25 approx.).

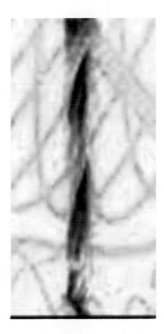

Figure 6.1 Multi-coloured thread for stitching (×25 approx.).

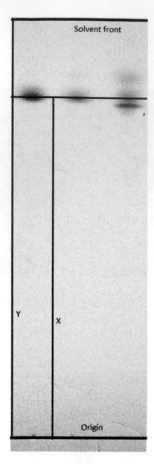

Figure 7.1 A typical thin line chromatography plate showing the separation of ink components. Each component has its own separation factor, known as R_f, which is calculated by dividing the distance the component has migrated (X) by the distance travelled by the solvent (Y).

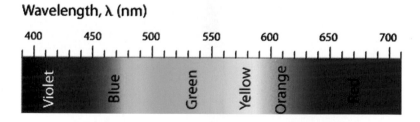

Figure 8.1 The electromagnetic spectrum.

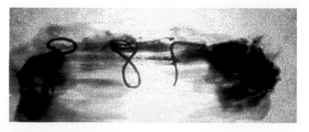

Figure 8.6 An entry covered with correction fluid viewed from behind the document illuminated with transmitted light.

5
The Examination of Printed Documents

5.1 Introduction

Traditionally, machine-produced documents fell into two separate categories: those produced in the office or home environment with machines capable of being used by most people with a minimal amount of knowledge as to how to operate them; and second, professional printing machines that typically would be located at a printworks dedicated to the production of high quality and usually large volumes of printed documentation ranging from letterheads to magazines. Into the former category, items such as typewriters, computer printers and photocopiers would fall (see Chapter 4). Into the latter category machines such as letterpress and offset lithographic printing presses would fall, which will be the focus of this chapter.

The distinction between 'amateur' and 'professional' printing of documents has become less marked. The computer and associated technological changes have tended to bring the two categories towards one another such that they now overlap significantly. For example, laser and inkjet printers are often to be found in a printworks and offset lithography presses can be scaled down into office machines for those wanting such devices (a trend that has largely been halted by the inkjet and laser printer).

Nonetheless, traditional printing techniques are still widely used and in this chapter some of the most frequently encountered processes will be described (Bruno, 2000) and related to the appearance of the printed product when viewed by the document examiner. This will make clear what features of a printed document can be determined when considering counterfeit and altered documents, especially those that are of particular importance in society such as currency and passports.

Foundations of Forensic Document Analysis: Theory and Practice, First Edition. Michael Allen.
© 2016 John Wiley & Sons, Ltd. Published 2016 by John Wiley & Sons, Ltd.
Companion Website: www.wiley.com/go/allen/forensicanalysis

5.2   Some general principles of printing

Whatever printing process is used to produce a document, a number of general issues will often apply, such as the properties of the inks that are used, how different colours are produced and how to reproduce images (as opposed to text) without applying such large amounts of ink to the paper that it will soak in and spoil the product.

5.2.1   Ink properties

Ink properties will vary depending on the print process used and on the substrate that is being printed on, be it paper, plastic, metal or some other material. Some general considerations might include: the viscosity (thickness) of the ink – since if it is too thin it will have a tendency to run but if too thick it may stick to the print surface and not the substrate; the drying properties of the ink – because if it dries too slowly printed sheets must be kept apart to avoid ink transferring from one sheet to another, but if it dries too quickly it might dry on the print plate before being printed onto the paper; its properties once printed – as the printed product may need to last for many years and air and light may tend to degrade the ink over time. Because of such factors, printing inks are complex chemical formulations (see Box 5.1).

Box 5.1 Printing ink composition

Printing inks need to have a number of properties for them to fulfil their function (Kunjappu, 2003). Printing inks impart colour by pigments rather than dyes. Pigments are insoluble whereas dyes are soluble. Pigments can be either organic (based on carbon molecules) or inorganic. One important factor that has caused changes in the pigments used is their toxicity. For example, lead (Pb) based pigments are not used now due to concerns over lead poisoning.

Because pigments are insoluble, they consist of microscopic particles suspended in a liquid. The size of the particles determines the intensity of the colour once the ink dries.

The thickness, or viscosity, of the ink reflects the different printing processes available. The viscosity is controlled by adding various polymer-based additives to the ink. Another important property of a printing ink is its drying speed, since if the ink takes a long time to dry this means handling the printed product carefully to avoid smudging. The drying of ink has a number of factors associated with it, including the absorption of the ink into the substrate (such as paper) and the reaction of the ink's components with the air.

5.2.2 Colour management

Colour reproduction in printing is typically achieved using a colour combination usually abbreviated to CMYK which is a mix of cyan (a shade of blue), yellow, magenta (a reddish pink) and black (sometimes referred to as the key – hence the initial K). A perfect combination of cyan, yellow and magenta should in theory produce black, but in reality their combination tends to produce a dark grey, so to produce black (typically needed for text) the black ink is used to give a darker printed product using just one ink.

The CMYK is often called a subtractive colour model and requires the inks to be at least semi-transparent so that when the inks overlap they combine (as opposed to the second ink blocking out the first ink applied). By this means, cyan and magenta interact to produce blue, magenta and yellow produce red, and cyan and yellow produce green. Shade variations will depend on the relative amounts of the CMYK colours present.

Depending on what is being printed, the management of the ink colours can vary. For example, if a company letterhead is being produced using perhaps just one particular corporate colour then that ink can be specially made up and used on its own instead of being produced using a corresponding CMYK combination.

5.2.3 Registration

If printing requires the use of more than one colour, then separate printing plates have to be produced for each colour. It is then crucial that the printed details that are printed sequentially using the different colours line up properly otherwise the finished product will not be of a suitable quality. This alignment process is called registration. In addition, if a document is printed on both sides (such as currency or passports), the registration can be used to add a feature to the document so that when either side is viewed separately the pattern of printing in the area has no obvious image content but when held up to the light the printing on the two sides is simultaneously visible to reveal the intended image as can be found in a number of banknotes (See Figure 5.1).

5.2.4 Half tone printing

If an image is to be printed, the amount of ink that would need to be applied to create a solid image may be in excess of what the paper substrate can absorb. Halftone printing gets around this by converting the image into a series of dots of varying size and varying separation between dots (Figure 5.2). Large, closely spaced dots will give the illusion of a dark, solid colour, whereas smaller and more widely separated dots will give the illusion of a solid but paler colour. It is only when viewed under low power magnification that it becomes apparent that the image is not solid at all but is made up of many dots.

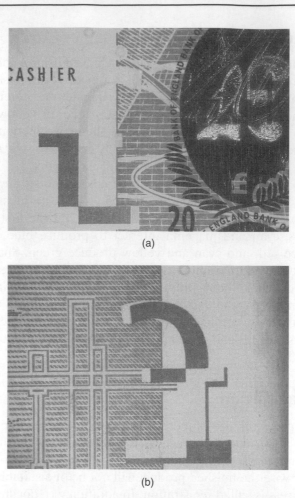

(a)

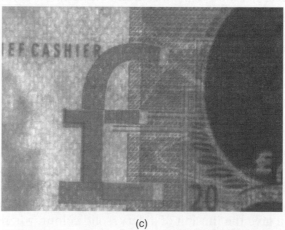

(b)

(c)

Figure 5.1 (a) The symbol on the front of the currency note; (b) the symbol on the reverse of the currency note; (c) the currency note viewed with transmitted light giving the completed symbol (x4 approx.). *(See insert for colour representation of the figure.)*

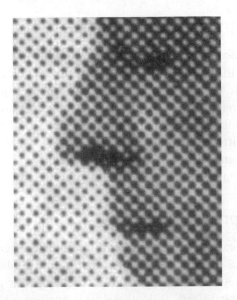

Figure 5.2 Close up of a half tone image showing how shades of grey are created by different densities of printed dots (x30 approx.).

The general principles of printing can be applied using a variety of printing techniques. Printing has changed a lot in recent times with the introduction of computer-based systems replacing more traditional techniques that used more conventional plate production and photographic methods. In the following sections some of the more widely encountered printing methods are described.

5.2.5 Traditional photographic and modern computer-based processes

Traditionally, printing involved manual processes, such as setting the letters of text or carving an image, which in time were overtaken by photographic processes after their discovery in the nineteenth century. With the advent of computers, their enhanced capability to manipulate text and images and the lower costs associated with reduced skilled manpower mean they are increasingly used. As far as the document examiner is concerned, the examination of all aspects of traditionally printing material was part of the scope of their expertise, but computers have become so complex that the examination of them has become a whole new discipline of digital forensics in its own right.

Notwithstanding considerable technological changes in printing technology, traditional printing techniques are still used, albeit often controlled in part by computers. There are a number of printing methods used and these will now be considered in turn.

5.3   Relief printing processes

Relief printing processes use a print plate in which the printing surface is above (in relief) the background, non-printing surface (Figure 5.3). The first devices to use relief printing were letterpress machines, which have a long history going back to the earliest machine-printed bibles produced by Johannes Gutenberg in fifteenth-century Germany and William Caxton in London soon after. Subsequent development of the basic method led to improvements and eventually such machines were widely used in the newspaper industry in particular.

5.3.1   Letterpress

In letterpress, the text or images were traditionally arranged in a frame called a form and once all of the required elements were in place they could then be inked and printed onto the substrate, typically paper (Bruno, 2000). The contact between the raised and inked print surface and the paper would occur under some pressure to ensure good transfer of the ink onto the paper. This contact had consequences for the appearance of the print on the paper. The ink would tend to be squeezed out around the edges of the relief characters leading to a halo of ink around the character – so-called ink squash (Figure 5.4). In addition, the applied pressure would often lead to the relief printing surface being demonstrably impressed into the paper surface.

The two features of ink squash and an impression on the paper surface can best be viewed under low power magnification and illuminated with an oblique light source to show the indentation.

A variant of letterpress is flexography, which uses a flexible print plate made from a light-sensitive plastic. Using a photographic film negative and ultraviolet light, the plastic hardens the surface of the plate where it is exposed to the light and the remaining surface areas are softer and can be washed away. A modern variant is to use a computer-guided laser to

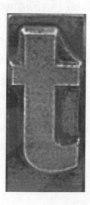

Figure 5.3   A letterpress printing surface (x25 approx.).

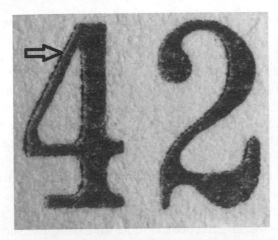

Figure 5.4 Ink squash around the edge of printed characters (x25 approx.). *(See insert for colour representation of the figure.)*

etch the surface of a flexible plastic print plate. Whatever method is used, the end result is similar, producing a flexible plastic sheet that has the print details in relief. Because it is flexible, it can be placed around a cylinder, inked and brought into contact with the paper under some pressure created by pressing up against a roller. Flexography has many commercial uses due to the flexible nature of the print plate, which allows it to be used on many different substrates such as cardboard packaging and plastic bags.

The even deposition of ink onto the printing plate is achieved by using an anilox roller that has a ceramic (pottery-like) surface covered by millions of small dimple-like depressions, or cells, of uniform spacing and depth. Ink applied to the anilox roller will fill the cells, which then can deliver a constant and consistent amount of ink to the print plate.

5.3.2 Stamp impressions

Stamping devices can come in a variety of constructions and be made from an assortment of materials. They all work by having a raised print surface which is inked and impressed onto the substrate, typically paper. Stamps can be used, for example, to put a date of receipt onto a document, to provide evidence of authorisation, or to apply a reference number to a document (such as the serial numbers found on currency or passports).

The stamp surface is usually either metal or a more flexible rubber-like material with the latter being made by a moulding process. Depending on the inks used and the degree of force applied, stampmarks made by such stamps often show ink squash and an impression into the paper surface.

Some stamping machines are highly automated (such as those used to add the serial number to currency) and produce stampmarks of regular appearance in terms of positioning on the document and the amount of ink applied. However, stamps can be applied by hand and in such cases the application may vary from one occasion to another in terms of both the pressure applied and also the evenness of application – if the stamp is twisted slightly, parts of the print surface may make better contact with the paper than others, resulting in an uneven application of ink. The majority of hand stamps are made of flexible material and this can 'give' when applied to the paper surface with some force (Figure 5.5). Eventually, the material of the stamp may break and deteriorate in a manner reminiscent of the way that single element typefaces get damaged (see Section 4.4 in Chapter 4).

Damage to a stamp (due to wear and tear after manufacture of the stamp) can have forensic value since it is likely to be unique. Even if a number of hand stamps were made at the same time each from the same mould, damage caused by such random effects, over time and with use, show up as minor imperfections distinguishing one from another. However, if there is an imperfection in the moulds used at the manufacturing stage, this will be reproduced on all stamps made using that mould and hence it will be a form of class defect.

Some stamps consist of an invariable design, such as a company logo. However, some stamps have variable elements, such as a series of moveable bands with numerals, months and years to enable a date to be stamped onto a document. Such moveable parts of the stamp can also yield forensic evidence if they are out of alignment, for example. But caution is needed when interpreting such evidence since there may be some variability due to the design of the stamp in the relative positioning of the moveable parts.

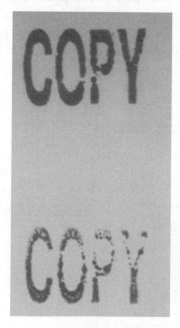

Figure 5.5 Stamp impressions vary in appearance depending on different conditions of applying. The upper stamp impression has been applied more heavily than the lower impression. *(See insert for colour representation of the figure.)*

One form of stamp that may also occur in cases is the pricing gun used usually in smaller stores to individually price items for sale. It too may become defective with heavy use and allow stolen goods to be traced back to the store from which they were taken, for example.

In some very busy finance departments, in order to save a particular person from signing their name on numerous occasions, a stamp of their signature may be made and used to authorise appropriate documents. Clearly, there needs to be controlled access to such a stamp, but it may be possible to copy a signature stamp or indeed any other stampmark. A photographic process is usually used to produce stamps, so a photo of a genuine stampmark can be used to produce copies. However, such copies will not be as true to the original since they are derived from an inked version on paper which is likely to lack the definition of detail of the original.

One last variant on relief printing using stampmarks is the seal used to make an impression in wax that even today may still be used on some official documents. Signature-based seals, known as chops, are still widely used in some areas of the world, particularly in parts of Asia. Detecting forged seals may require complex computer image comparisons using various mathematical algorithms to analyse the images of genuine and suspect stampmarks (Lee et al., 2012).

5.4 Planographic printing

In the relief printing processes discussed in the previous section, the printing surface is above the background non-printing areas (Bruno, 2000). In planographic printing, the printing and non-printing areas are in the same plane. The two areas are distinguished not by differing topology but by differing chemical properties. Lithography (the term is derived from the Greek for stone writing) has been around in various forms for a very long time, but in modern times it is most frequently encountered as offset lithography (often just referred to as offset). Printing plates are typically made from thin aluminium and they have a surface coating that reacts to light. In the presence of light (corresponding to the printing area) the surface becomes hydrophobic (water repelling, oil attracting) and the non-printing area is hydrophilic (water attracting, oil repelling). The printing inks used are oil based and are attracted to the image area and away from the hydrophobic non-printing areas.

Printing is often done using CMYK but can also be done using bespoke coloured inks. The inked plates are brought into contact with a rubber (or similar material) blanket (typically wound around a cylinder) and the ink is thereby transferred from the printing plate to the blanket – a process known as offsetting. The ink is then transferred from the blanket to the paper. The reason for offsetting is so that the ink is released from a more flexible material which makes better contact with the paper than would the flat printing plate. (In relief printing, good contact between the print surface and paper is ensured with the application of some pressure – see previous section.)

Figure 5.6   The gradual merging of colours found in split duct printing. *(See insert for colour representation of the figure.)*

Because of the planographic process, it is possible to set up an offset printing press with two inks that will merge gradually into one another. For example yellow and blue inks may be used that gradually merge giving yellow then pale green, darker green and then blue inking across a document. This is often referred to as split duct printing (Figure 5.6) (or rainbow printing) and the result is difficult to copy by counterfeiters.

5.5   Recess printing

Recess printing uses print plates in which the image is below that of the non-printing area – in other words the complete opposite to relief printing processes such as letterpress – see Section 5.3. Recess printing processes are often called intaglio processes (Bruno, 2000).

The means by which the recesses are created can vary – traditionally the plate might be engraved (manually cut away – a print process known as gravure) or etched (using strong acid, for example, to eat into a metal plate surface) but increasingly automated processes are used, such as laser engraving of metal plates. The quality of the image produced by highly skilled engravers can be very high with very fine detail as might be found, for example, on banknotes and passports. These fine details are extremely difficult to copy by counterfeiters and constitute a security feature of a document. The depth and width of the engraved areas will determine the amount of ink that will fill the recesses, which in turn will affect the amount of ink on the paper. Because the non-printing area is above the ink, it is necessary to make sure that it is free from any traces of ink, and this is achieved by the presence of a so-called doctor blade that wipes across the plate surface to remove any residual ink.

The ink used in recess printing is very viscous (thick) since it has to be pulled out of the recess onto the paper under some pressure. Because the ink is so thick and because the amount of ink can be varied by altering the dimensions of the recess, recess printing methods are capable of producing very high quality images in terms of the depth of coloration achieved. The ink is so viscous that it will usually sit on the surface of the paper substrate (Figure 5.7),

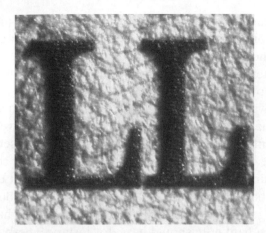

Figure 5.7 Close up showing raised ink on paper surface from a recessed printing process viewed under oblique lighting (x25 approx.). *(See insert for colour representation of the figure.)*

giving it a tactile effect that can be readily detected just by touching with a finger tip to feel the presence of the thick ink. This tactile quality is a security feature of this printing process that is often used in certain types of important documents such as currency and passports.

5.6 Screen printing

In screen printing the ink is forced through a fine mesh using a squeegee device and the non-printing areas are represented by a stencil on the mesh that prevents the ink transfer through the mesh (Bruno, 2000). Inks of a variety of types can be used depending to some extent on the nature of the substrate, which can vary from paper to cloth to plastics and many other materials. In addition the substrate need not be planar but rather can be shaped, such as a bottle. It is rarely encountered on documents in casework but it may be relevant to an examination of counterfeit packing of pirated goods, for example. Because of the mesh through which the ink is forced, magnification shows a stepped cell-like appearance of the ink. If several colours are to be used, they are printed sequentially and this requires good registration of the printed images.

5.7 Security documents

The printing techniques described above are some of the main categories typically encountered in forensic casework. Printing, like any other business, runs along mainly commercial lines. In practice, this means that the processes used are partly dictated by cost for a given quality of product. However, there is another important dimension to many documents that occur in forensic contexts, namely – how easy is it to copy or alter a genuine document?

Important documents involved in financial transactions (such as cheques and banknotes) or documents that give entitlement (such as passports and identity cards) should be made in such a way as to make them difficult to counterfeit or alter. In addition, access to the production processes from the original designs to the printing plates, inks and papers used need to be tightly controlled to prevent unauthorised access. Documents such as passports also have to be personalised when issued and the processes involved with that must also be tightly controlled to ensure that the final product is secure and there is a minimal chance of either tampering with it or completely counterfeiting it.

Preventing counterfeiting is only possible in the context of the person or machine that it has to fool. For this reason, counterfeit detection is often regarded as a staged process. A member of the public may have some notion of what features a banknote should have, for instance, perhaps aware that it might show up some distinctive details under ultraviolet light. Border security staff will have special training to detect suspect passports and identity cards often based on a rapid assessment of the document. The provision of detailed expert forensic evidence will then fall to those with the highest level of expertise to describe and explain to a court, for example, the reasons why a document is genuine or otherwise based on a detailed knowledge of the materials and processes used and their significance to a particular case situation. A counterfeit is less and less likely to fool those with the greater training and expertise.

The security of a document can be enhanced in a variety of ways. Starting with the design of the document, it is the case that the more intricate and involved the images that are to be printed, the more difficult it will be to copy. Any copying process, be it photographic or electronic scanning, will inevitably lead to a loss of image quality. The ways in which documents can be counterfeited must therefore be borne in mind at the design stage since, for example, colour photocopiers are readily available and it would not be a very secure document that could be convincingly copied simply using a colour copier. The choice of colours and design detail can make colour copying more difficult by exploiting the copier's inability to reproduce very fine detail and certain colours (especially some lighter, pastel shades) as clearly as on an original document.

Once the design has been finalised, the materials (paper and ink) and printing processes used to produce the document will in turn help to make it difficult to counterfeit. First the paper itself can be made secure (see Chapter 6). Most readily available paper contains optical brighteners to make the paper appear brighter (especially when viewed under ultraviolet light when the paper glows white) than it otherwise would. Paper that does *not* contain optical brighteners is not so easily obtained (such papers appear a dull purplish when viewed under ultraviolet light). To make the paper more secure, a watermark will certainly be created at the paper manufacturing stage. Watermarks vary in quality, ranging from a relatively simple design seen as grey against white when viewed with transmitted light to more complex designs that show tonal variation in the pattern. The latter watermarks are produced on cylinder mould paper, which is less readily available and is the result of a complex paper-making process.

Watermarks have been used in paper manufacture for a long time but remain one of the most effective anti-counterfeiting measures available. Introducing a watermark into paper after it has been manufactured is essentially impossible so counterfeiters can only attempt to create the appearance of a watermark being present.

The position of a watermark on a document can be made to coincide with particular areas of the document so that the viewing of the watermark is unhindered by obscuring ink. In a multi-page document such as a passport, it is possible to put different watermarks onto various pages thus further adding to the task of the counterfeiter. In banknotes it is possible to add a security thread that is woven into the paper at the time of manufacture. This process is again virtually impossible to re-create so the counterfeiter can only produce something that looks right but is in fact incorrectly constructed. The threads can have sophisticated details printed on them, such as inks having particular optical properties and microprinting – which, as its name suggests, is very small but high-quality printed detail barely legible and visible to the naked eye (Figure 5.8) but which, when copied, loses its distinct character forms and tends to become an illegible blur.

The printing processes used to produce security documents are essentially mainstream traditional printing techniques but they are of a very high quality and use inks of particular formulations, the components of which may impart particular properties to the ink that the counterfeiter cannot reproduce (see also Chapter 6). Some inks appear to change colour when viewed at different

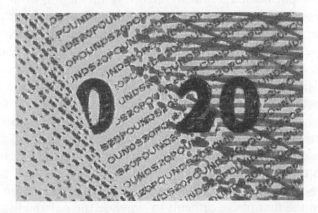

Figure 5.8 Microprinting (x25 approx.). *(See insert for colour representation of the figure.)*

angles (optically variable inks); some inks have particular properties when viewed under ultraviolet light; and some inks have a pearl-like appearance (pearlescent inks). These properties are imparted by the complex materials present in the ink formulation.

Even relatively simple ideas can make counterfeiting difficult, such as printing details on each side of a sheet of paper which, when viewed with transmitted light shone through the document, make a particular pattern. Documents that have a serial number, such as passports and currency, typically have the number printed using letterpress. The numbers can be further embellished by using different coloured inks for the numerals, as can be found on a £20 note. Of course a serial number is intended to be unique to a given banknote and so the forger can either attempt to give each counterfeit a different serial number or, more commonly, a series of counterfeits will all have the same serial number.

5.7.1   Personalisation of documents

Documents that require the addition of details onto them are potentially vulnerable to misuse. If document production is securely controlled then access to blank documents should be difficult for unauthorised people. The addition of details nonetheless needs to also be done in such a way as to minimise the likelihood of someone being able to issue a fraudulently personalised, genuinely printed, document such as a passport or identity card.

Traditionally, personalisation was relatively crude in many cases, such as the manual typing in of information and the use of glue to stick in a passport-sized photograph that was endorsed by a signature across the photo to demonstrate its authenticity! Standards for the quality of modern security documents have improved immeasurably (although the rate of improvement does vary across the world) in recent times and the personalisation process is significantly more sophisticated, typically involving the digital printing processes that were described in the previous chapter, particularly laser printing and inkjet printing. In addition, the photographic image may be printed securely onto the page and many such documents have the biographical page laminated so as to reduce the ease with which the details can subsequently be tampered with. The laminates are made of clear plastic and they usually consist of several layers that are bonded together making it very difficult to separate the layers one from another and from the paper of the document itself. Some of the layers can have special properties, such as the capability of being etched by a laser beam to, for example, include an image of the document holder derived from their passport photo.

Documents can, therefore, be made so as to make them difficult to counterfeit in the first place, difficult to simulate the personalisation process successfully and secured to make tampering as difficult as possible. Despite all of these safeguards, there is an industry in both counterfeiting and altering documents that forms a significant challenge to the legal movement of people around the world and for this reason the authorities responsible for the production and administration of these important documents are constantly adding new and more sophisticated barriers designed to reduce yet further the misuse of such documents. As part of that endeavour, the paper itself makes a significant contribution to a document's security, and in the next chapter the manufacture of paper will be described.

5.8 Dry transfer lettering

Dry transfers are generally available as plastic backing sheets from which letters, numbers, symbols and other material can be transferred, usually to paper, by rubbing over the area of the sheet with a pen or some similar implement. This causes the character to be transferred onto the paper, thus leaving a gap on the backing sheet where the character was originally. They are used particularly in the production of artwork for various purposes. Many different font styles and sizes are available.

Dry transfers have been used in a number of case types that either require anonymity of the sender or else because they have a printed appearance, superficially at least, they can be used to replace some erased printed material on a document.

If dry transfers have been used on a suspect document and if sheets of dry transfers have been recovered from a suspect, then there may well be a request that a comparison be made to see if the recovered sheets were used to produce the document in question. The first step is essentially the same as with a type-script comparison, namely to make sure that the font style and size used on the document is the same as that on the sheet. Assuming it is, then the letters, numbers and any other relevant symbols that are missing from the sheet can be compared to those present on the document. The evidence available at this stage can be very strong if the particular characters missing from the sheet coincide exactly with the characters present on the suspect document. Of course this does depend on the extent of the coincidence. If just one letter E is missing from the sheet and just one letter E dry transfer is on the document then this could be a chance occurrence. But as more and more characters are transferred, the likelihood of an exact coincidental match decreases.

Occasionally, the transfer process is imperfect, leading to a partial transfer of a character. This provides potentially excellent evidence to link a transfer sheet to transfers on a page if the two partial transfers can be shown to have originally been part of the same character.

Another aspect can be examined, which is the transfer process carried out by the application of pressure from a pen or similar implement (Welch, 1986). In particular, some of the adhesive material that holds the transfer in place

Table 5.1   Diagnostic features of printing processes.

Printing feature	Possibilities
Impression in surface of paper	<ul><li>Letterpress – will also show ink squash</li><li>Typewriter</li><li>Impact matrix printer – characters made of separate dots</li></ul>
Toner	<ul><li>Laser printer</li><li>Photocopier</li></ul>
Raised ink deposit	<ul><li>Recess printing method such as gravure/intaglio</li></ul>
Ink soaked into paper, no impression	<ul><li>Inkjet – discrete dots of (usually) the four colours cyan, yellow, magenta and black</li><li>Offset lithography – often identified when other methods have been discounted as fairly featureless</li></ul>
Sawtooth edge to characters	<ul><li>Silk screen – ink present</li><li>Fax – often heat sensitive paper so no ink present</li></ul>
Waxy appearance	<ul><li>Thermal ink</li></ul>

on its backing sheet is transferred with the transfer itself and this may show a pattern of pen movements on the document when viewed under an ultraviolet light source which can be compared to the pattern on the sheet.

5.9   Key diagnostic features of various printing methods

In Chapters 4 and 5 a variety of different methods of printing were described. Table 5.1 summarises some of the key features that can be used to determine the method of printing used on a document of unknown origin.

5.10   Case notes in printing cases

Generally, the first step when examining a questioned printed document is to determine the process(es) used to produce it. Often there is specimen genuine material to compare it with and typically a counterfeit document will not have been produced using the same processes as a genuine document nor will the questioned document have been produced to the same standard as the genuine one. This is a reflection of the quality of the equipment and materials that are usually available to, and employed by, official (typically government) authorities rather than to the counterfeiter.

Identification of the print process, and the observations leading to it, must be noted. It is a good idea to note not only the positive observations but also the negative ones, such as an absence of indentation (thus making letterpress unlikely) or the absence of a thick ink deposit (thus making gravure unlikely). The reasoning behind this approach is that some printing processes, particularly offset lithography, tend to produce a printed product that has few characteristic features.

Obviously the notes made reflect the nature of the examination being undertaken. If, for example, the issue is how a questioned document has been printed and whether it is it genuine, then identifying the print processes involved may effectively complete the examination. However, in cases where there is suspected to be a particular source for the questioned documents, there may be a need to compare the printing on a number of suspect documents to determine whether or not they share a common source and to determine whether they have been produced using equipment and materials at a particular location (such as at a particular printworks). In these cases it is necessary to examine the printing with a view to identifying features that may link them, such as defects and imperfections (often microscopic) of the printed documents (similar in some ways to defects found on laser printed or photocopied documents) which recur from one to another showing that they share a common source. Notes must be made showing where these occur, for example on a photocopy of the document, so that they can be used as evidence.

If items such as printing plates or photographic images (artwork) are available for examination, then the same principles apply, namely detecting any characteristic features to link the images on the items with the printed documents. Any evidence found must be recorded clearly in the notes by whatever method is most convenient, with photographs or annotated photocopies often being ideal.

Printing ink and paper may be recovered from suspect premises but the forensic evidence is often limited from such items unless there is something characteristic about them. Often, the paper and ink used are readily available and as such are less likely to be distinctive. Nonetheless, notes should be made as to the nature of such materials even if little evidence of value accrues from their examination.

The combined value of the observations in the case in relation to the question being asked will then determine which findings are more (or less) relevant and hence inform a conclusion that is appropriately weighted given various possible explanations for the findings.

5.11   Reports in cases involving printing

Cases in this category often involve pieces of equipment, processes and materials with which the non-expert is less familiar (although of course the many printed products, ranging from newsprint to packaging, are familiar). For this reason, the expert's report may need to include some brief background information about the relevant printing processes being considered so the reader can put into context the expert's findings and conclusions. As with all reports it is ideal to avoid use of jargon terms, but if they have to be used a brief explanation of their meaning can be appended in a suitable way to help the reader.

Most printing cases fall into one (or both) of two main categories: (i) is the suspect document genuine or a counterfeit and (ii) how was the suspect document printed and (sometimes) was it printed using the particular equipment at a given place (such as a suspect's printworks)? The purpose of the forensic examination in a case can be set out according to these terms and thus any findings and conclusions can then be related to this purpose.

The findings that are central to cases of this type are often amenable to photographic records and these can be incorporated into a report to show each point as it is described in the report. It is a good idea to describe each feature of the printed document one at a time and to show photographs that will assist the reader to fully understand their significance.

As with any complex report, a brief summary describing the conclusions in the absence of explanatory findings will make it clear to the reader what the expert's opinion is.

Printing examination: a worked example

In this section, an example of how to approach a case and make notes is demonstrated. The worked example is intended to show a general process in terms of thinking and doing, rather than with the expectation that the reader will 'test' themselves to see if they can get the 'right' answer (although getting the 'right' answer could be regarded as a welcome bonus!).

It should be stressed that there are a number of different ways to make notes and the intention here is to show the kinds of issues that need to be considered and how these interrelate with the observation process leading to a conclusion.

Case circumstances

A suspected counterfeit banknote is submitted for examination.

Purpose

To determine whether or not the submitted banknote is counterfeit and to establish how it has been produced.

In addition, the investigator wants an indication of the quality of the counterfeit. The reason is that if it is obviously so poor that no reasonable person would accept it as a genuine banknote, then the perpetrator might argue that it was not done to deceive but for some other reason (such as 'for fun'.)

Items submitted

Item 1: Banknote

Case notes

Observations	Thoughts
A genuine banknote with security features such as those listed will be immediately apparent by the high quality materials and printing processes used. The various security features should all be checked.	What materials and printing processes should be used in a genuine banknote of this type?
While the absence of a watermark, for example, in the submitted note would on its own provide compelling evidence of counterfeiting, it is best to make detailed observations and to note down all of the features so that undue reliance is not placed on just one difference from a genuine banknote.	This will vary between banknotes of different values and from different countries. If the banknote is unfamiliar it is necessary to obtain a genuine banknote as a specimen. In this case, the banknote is familiar and should contain a number of security features such as: • UV dull paper with UV-reactive fibres, • watermark of correct design, • some details printed intaglio, • bulk of detail printed offset lithography, • microprinting, • security thread.
In this case, none of the security features that are to be found in a genuine specimen banknote of the relevant kind are present in the submitted banknote.	

At this point, the conclusion that the banknote submitted is a counterfeit is fully justified. The next part of the examination is to determine how the counterfeit has been produced. Traditionally, counterfeit currency was often produced using machines and processes mainly available to professional printers. However, modern printworks may have both traditional machinery and computer-based printers, such as those described in Chapter 4, available and such devices are of course easily available to the wider public.

Observations	Thoughts
When viewed under the microscope, the printing of the banknote is all offset lithography with the exception of the serial number, which has been stamped on (as shown by the impression into the paper and ink squash) but the font style of the numbering differs from that of the specimen. A simulated watermark has been printed on using a pale cream ink. The paper is UV-bright. All differences between a genuine banknote and item 1 need to be documented in the notes and preferably photographed.	These observations run against much of the current trend of using digital printers, such as a colour laser printer, when producing counterfeit security documents. The use of offset lithography suggests the possibility that the submitted banknote has been produced at a printworks.

When determining how a counterfeit has been produced, an often unasked question, but an important question nonetheless, is whether it might be possible to find evidential links between the counterfeit document and machines or materials from a printworks *if one was identified at some point in the future.*

Observations	Thoughts
The printing shows a number of small imperfections in the detail which might be apparent if the printing plate or even the offset blanket were examined. The numbers of the serial number appear to be undamaged.	If a printworks were to become the focus of the investigation then retrieval of such items as the printing plates or possibly artwork or computer images *could* provide a link between the counterfeit and the place where it was printed.
The print quality is not as good as a genuine note and the paper does not have the necessary qualities. But it could have been much cruder.	Is the counterfeit of such a quality as to deceive? At one extreme, a black and white photocopy would be unconvincing. At the other extreme, a much more sophisticated counterfeit could be produced with unlimited resources. Overall, item 1 is not a bad attempt and the simulated watermark suggests this is more than just someone 'having a go'.

Report of Forensic Expert

(Again, it is stressed that this report is intended to demonstrate an approach and not to be a test of getting the 'right' answer.)

Qualifications and experience ...

Scope of expertise ...

Items examined

I have examined the following items at the instruction of (the investigating authority). They were received at the laboratory on (dates).

Item 1: Banknote

Purpose

I have examined the banknote, item 1, with a view to determining whether or not it is a counterfeit. In addition I have determined both the method and quality of production of item 1.

Findings

The banknote, item 1, differs from specimen banknotes of this type in a number of significant respects. For example, the type of paper used, the absence of a genuine watermark in the paper and the printing processes used all differ those of a specimen banknote. However, item 1 does bear a simulated watermark and the overall quality of the printing is good.

[It is often a good idea to insert relevant photographs here to further illustrate the nature of the differences being described.]

I conclude that the banknote, item 1, is not a genuine banknote but is a counterfeit. With the exception of the serial numbers, item 1 has been printed using a process called offset lithography which is usually encountered in printworks and not in domestic locations. The serial number has been printed using letterpress, possibly using a metal stamping device.

The quality of printing and the presence of a simulated watermark in item 1 suggest that this is a reasonably good attempt to produce a convincing counterfeit banknote.

Summary

Item 1 is a counterfeit banknote.

As to the possible comparison to materials recovered from a suspect printworks at some time in the future, this is best explained in a letter to the investigator since it is not at present part of the evidence but rather constitutes advice as to what might be possible to achieve.

References

Bruno, M. H. (2000). *Pocket Pal: A Graphic Arts Production Handbook* (18th edition) Graphic Arts Technical Foundation.

Kunjappu, J. (2003). Ink chemistry. *Chemistry in Britain*, 39(3), 22–25.

Lee, J., Kong, S. G., Lee, Y., et al. (2012). Forged seal detection based on the seal overlay metric. *Forensic Science International*, 214(1–3), 200–206. doi:10.1016/j.forsciint.2011.08.009.

Welch, J. R. (1986). The linking of a counterfeit document to individual sheets of dry-transfer lettering through the transfer of fluorescent glue. *Journal of the Forensic Science Society*, 26(4), 253–256. doi:10.1016/S0015-7368(86)72492-4.

6
Materials Used to Create Documents

Documents are increasingly being viewed electronically on computers and are moved around in cyberspace. But documents continue to exist in a real world of physical entities and it is necessary for the forensic document examiner to have a good knowledge of the materials from which documents are constructed. In this chapter, the materials and processes from which these physical objects are made will be described. However, the various analytical methods available for examining these materials will be considered in Chapter 7 and the casework context of alterations to documents will be described in Chapter 8.

Document examiners come from a variety of educational backgrounds, usually, but not always, with a strong scientific content. The examination of the materials present in a document can be carried out at a number of levels reflecting factors such as time available for the examination, costs, equipment availability and the expertise of the expert or their colleagues. It is to be expected that as the scientific complexity of an examination increases, the feasibility of carrying out these examinations decreases. For example, comparing two sheets of paper can be done at a straightforward level (such as size, colour, ruled markings), a more complex level (such as thickness measured using a micrometer to take an average of readings across a sheet or examination under differing ultraviolet wavelengths), or at an even more complex level (such as determining the plant material from which the paper is made by high power microscopy, requiring an associated high level of botanical knowledge).

In this chapter, the physical elements from which documents are made will be described and the general approach to their examination will be shown.

Foundations of Forensic Document Analysis: Theory and Practice, First Edition. Michael Allen.
© 2016 John Wiley & Sons, Ltd. Published 2016 by John Wiley & Sons, Ltd.
Companion Website: www.wiley.com/go/allen/forensicanalysis

Increasingly complex methods may simply be unavailable to the expert and, in any event, may be unnecessary if other, simpler techniques are sufficient. In general, the examination strategy tends to go from simple to complex and at the same time from non-destructive to destructive, from cheap to expensive and requiring increasingly specialist equipment and knowledge. In addition, showing that two physical objects – be they paper, ink or some other component of a document – are different is generally much easier than showing they are similar since in the latter situation there is always the possibility that 'just one more (complex and expensive) test' might show a difference. Further, since two objects cannot logically be one and the same object, there will always be some differences between any two 'similar' objects and hence the degree of similarity will always need to be determined when explaining its significance.

Examination strategies of the physical components of a document will therefore vary from case to case and from laboratory to laboratory. ASTM (formerly the American Society for Testing and Materials) in the USA has published standard approaches to examining the materials from which documents are created and these will be given in the relevant sections below. These standards are recommendations of good practice but in a given case they may need to be interpreted flexibly depending on the materials and resources available.

6.1   Paper

By far the most common substrate for a document is traditional paper. However, handwriting can occur on an almost limitless number of other materials such as graffiti on all manner of buildings, on fabric (such as the inside of a sports bag), on CDs and DVDs and so on.

Historically, handwriting was often written on other paper-like materials. One such is parchment made from animal skins such as goat or sheep or, when made from calf skin, known as vellum.

Paper is usually made from plant material, the main constituent of which is cellulose fibres. (Papyrus is made from parts of particular plants and its method of manufacture is generally different to that described below for modern paper.) The source of the fibres can vary from trees (by far the most commonly encountered) to grasses (may be used in some countries) and other materials such as cotton (specifically the hairs on the seeds for high quality papers) and bast fibres (certain botanical elements of plants such as hemp and jute). Individual fibres are typically about 3–5 mm in length and about 50 μ in diameter (1000 μ being the same as 1 mm). The basic requirement is that the fibres are processed in such a way as to produce a thin mat of overlapping fibres capable of receiving ink in a stable and long-term manner.

6.1.1 Manufacture of paper

In order to make paper, it is first necessary to create a pulp consisting mostly of water (it is for this reason that paper mills are situated near large sources of water) into which has been added the fibre material after it has been removed from the trees (or other vegetable matter) by a process of grinding down and chemical treatment. The latter treatment involves cooking the fibres in the presence of some strong chemicals that help to eliminate impurities from the pulp mixture, particularly lignin which tends to give paper a yellowish colour if left in the mix.

Paper of course has many uses and it depends on the intended use of the product as to how the basic paper formulation is treated. For example, paper that is intended for wrapping or paper bags needs to be reasonably physically strong but does not need to have a particularly pleasant appearance, whereas writing paper needs to be capable of taking ink onto its surface and it might be desirable that it be very white, while paper for currency needs to be very strong indeed to stay in circulation despite continuous handling and also needs to be secure against counterfeiting. For the various uses to which paper can be put, additives (see Section 6.1.2) will be put into the mix during manufacture to impart the desired properties.

The slurry-like pulp material forms the basic paper sheet through the removal the excess water leaving behind the paper fibres. There are two main processes used on an industrial scale to achieve this. They are known as the Fourdrinier process and the cylinder mould process.

In the Fourdrinier process, the pulp passes over a mesh, the so-called wire (today made out of plastic but historically from a metal wire), through which much of the water drains, leaving the fibres caught as a mat on the wire surface. The paper is still very moist at this stage but physically quite robust such that a watermark can be produced using a raised design on a cylinder (known as a dandy roll), which is pressed into the paper causing some fibres to be displaced in the area of the raised design and hence making the paper more translucent at that point. However, such watermarks tend not to be as good as those produced by the cylinder mould process (see below).

The wet mat of fibres needs to have almost all of the remaining water removed by pressing and heating it. In order to compact and make the paper surface smoother, it is then passed through heavy rollers (a process called calendering).

Cylinder mould paper machines are more rarely encountered and they are often used to produce security paper (for documents that are made more difficult to counterfeit). Paper is made on a revolving wire-covered cylinder that is partly immersed in a vat of paper pulp. A relief pattern on the mesh will impart a watermark to the paper as the fibres are less densely accumulated in these areas. The watermark produced can have a multi-tonal (shades of grey) appearance of great clarity and for this reason it is the manufacturing process of choice for many types of security documents as the watermark remains one of the most difficult properties of a sheet of paper to simulate.

6.1.2   Additives used in papermaking

The use for which particular paper products are made will determine the detailed manufacturing process used, including what additives are needed to give the paper its desired properties. The colour of paper is an obvious property and for many uses white paper is needed. Wood pulp tends to produce paper of an off-white appearance, so in order to improve its whiteness optical brighteners are often added. These chemicals have the property of absorbing ultraviolet light and re-emitting it in the blue part of the visible spectrum (see Box 8.1 in Chapter 8). This makes the paper appear brighter and whiter. When viewed under ultraviolet light, such papers are extremely bright whereas paper that does not contain optical brighteners will appear a dull violet colour.

Paper made from fibres only (no additives) will tend to have poor ink receptivity. In other words, an ink applied to the paper will tend to bleed into the fibres with unsatisfactory results. The particular ink that is to be used may be for writing purposes or printing purposes and the quality of the final product will be of importance to ensure satisfactory results. In order to make the paper more receptive to ink it is treated with a material called a sizing agent (Biermann, 1996). There are a number of such agents that can either be added to the paper while it is still wet (and hence the agent is dispersed throughout the sheet) or once the sheet has been dried and the agent is present on the paper surface only.

Fillers are added to the paper to make it smoother and to improve its optical qualities (since translucent paper is not usually ideal), effectively filling in the gaps between the paper fibres. Examples of fillers are clay and titanium dioxide, which are added at the pulp stage so that the fillers are present through the whole sheet.

Paper can be coated with a variety of further chemicals to impart various properties to it, such as a glossy finish, again depending on its intended use in, for example, a high quality brochure or catalogue.

6.1.3   Paper for security documents

The majority of security documents are produced on UV-dull paper as this is much less encountered in the wider commercial marketplace, and it is often made using the cylinder mould process with a high quality, tonal watermark. The production of such paper is expensive and tightly controlled to make it unavailable to unauthorised use. Additionally, coloured or ultraviolet fluorescent fibres can be added randomly to the paper as can planchettes (small, usually circular small pieces of coloured paper) to impart uniqueness to each sheet of paper produced.

Simulating security paper should be as difficult as possible for the counter-feiter as the value of the original document is undermined by easy copying. Simulating UV-dull paper may be done by printing a suitable material onto the surface of a piece of UV-bright paper, and likewise the appearance of a watermark can be attempted by printing onto the surface of a piece of paper in a pale cream ink to give the appearance of the correct watermark. Fibres and planchettes might also be printed on (but almost certainly the same fibre pattern will then be apparent on each simulated sheet) and it is not unknown for forgers to draw in fibres by hand!

6.1.4 Paper products

Paper can be the basis for other products apart from sheets of paper. The paper is the main constituent of the product but it is processed in various ways to create something more than just a piece of paper.

6.1.4.1 Envelopes Envelopes are nearly always made from paper although some may be made from plastics when there is a need for excep-tional physical strength against tearing and damage. The paper from which an envelope is made can be examined in just the same way as for paper itself, but in addition the dimensions of the finished envelope, the method of construction, the adhesive used and any printing matter on the envelope (both on the outside surface and more commonly on the inside surface) can be used to differentiate between envelopes. It is common practice for envelope manufacturers to print various batch details or even dates of production on an inaccessible inner corner of the envelope, which can also help in either comparing or dating envelopes.

6.1.4.2 Passports Paper for security documents that consist of a single sheet of paper, such as currency or driving licences, has already been described. However, passports are somewhat different in that they require construction of a booklet from constituent pieces of paper and indeed other materials such as the cover and the thread used to sew the pages into the booklet. All aspects of the design of security documents are constantly being updated in line with technological changes. Even the thread used to sew up passports has become increasingly sophisticated, with several colours inter-twined (Figure 6.1) and some fluorescing under ultraviolet light, for example. The material used to produce the covers also will be tightly controlled so as not to be accessible to unauthorised users. Tampering with genuine passports can involve undoing the stitching and re-stitching to reform the passport. The stitching holes in the paper will often show evidence of widening as the thread is manipulated more than normal causing damage to the original stitch holes.

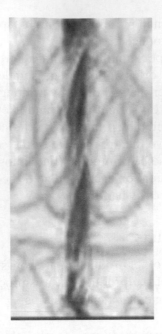

Figure 6.1   Multi-coloured thread for stitching (x25 approx.). *(See insert for colour representation of the figure.)*

Passport numbering has also become more involved with, for example, perforation of the whole passport with its unique reference number through all pages (Figure 6.2). This can be achieved mechanically or by using a laser beam. The end product in a genuine passport has a very clean appearance around the holes, whereas counterfeiters do not have access to the necessary equipment and so produce an inferior simulation.

6.1.4.3 Laminates   Laminates are plastic (polymer) based materials and as such are not, of course, paper products. However, they are widely used in security documents such as passports and identity cards. The personalising of passports and other security documents is usually done using digital

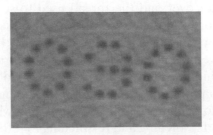

Figure 6.2   Perforated pages of a passport (x3 approx.).

technology as described in Chapter 4 (typically a laser printer), but the protection of that information from tampering has become more effective with the use of polymer laminates such as polycarbonates. These have become increasingly sophisticated, often made up of several layers, some of which, for example, can be engraved by a laser, some of which can contain yet more security devices such as holograms. Because of the importance of documents of this type, international standards are set to ensure that security documents can meet an adequate level of security that enables counterfeits to be identified with confidence.

6.2 Ink

Inks come in a variety of formulations depending on their use. The most commonly encountered in forensic document examination are pen inks, and in particular ballpoint pen inks, although other types, such as gel pen inks, are becoming more popular. Printing inks are used in many documents, but those of forensic interest tend to be security documents, where ink comparison per se is not the issue so much as determining whether the correct type of ink is present or whether an incorrect ink has been used as part of a simulation.

6.2.1 Pen inks

The methods of production and in particular the chemical composition of inks is often sensitive commercial information. However, in order to be satisfactory products, inks must comply with the needs for which they are made. Writing inks require a number of properties to be effective, such as the need to be colour-fast (that is they do not fade under normal circumstances, although many inks subjected to strong sunlight will fade given enough time), dry quickly on the page, and be delivered by the pen type concerned (such as a ballpoint pen or a fountain pen). As a result, inks contain a number of components that impart particular properties to them (Brunelle & Crawford, 2003). The all-important coloured component is made up from dyes (soluble colour) and pigments (insoluble colour).

A solvent is required to act as a vehicle for the other components of the ink. The solvent can be either water (for example in fountain pen inks) or organic (for example ballpoint pen inks). Ink has to flow from the writing implement onto the paper and this requires that the ink has the appropriate thickness (or viscosity), this is controlled by the presence of resins in the ink. Other components of the ink may be needed to control its surface properties once it is on the paper and emulsifiers can be added to ensure that any aqueous and non-aqueous components mix properly. Once the ink is on the paper it is important that it does not fade or react with the environment, so to reduce this the ink may contain antioxidants.

6.2.2　Printing inks

The mainstream, everyday printing of material such as magazines and pack-aging rarely requires special inks to be used. The inks used will have the nec-essary properties for the product being made.

Specialist inks are available for use in the production of security documents. The manufacture and distribution of such inks are likely to be more tightly controlled to avoid them getting into the hands of the counterfeiter. Examples of such inks are:

- Pearlescent inks, which have a shiny pearl-like appearance derived from the presence of flakes of refractive and reflective material suspended in the ink.

- Thermochromic inks that change colour with a change in temperature.

- Iridescent (optically variable) inks that change colour depending upon the angle at which they are viewed.

6.3　Staples

Occasionally a multipage document will be held together by means of staples, and if the source of such documents is called into question then it may be necessary to determine whether staples recovered from a suspect match those in question.

Staples are of two main kinds: those that are available commercially in pre-packed form; and those that are often used in the printing industry, where a length of metal is cut from a roll of wire and bent into a staple before being inserted into the document. Pre-packed staples come in a variety of different sizes and colours (some are silver coloured others more bronze coloured for example). The thickness of the wire from which the staple is made is an impor-tant factor in determining how many sheets of paper can be stapled. A staple made from a very thin wire would buckle if it was used to staple together too many sheets. On the other hand, a thicker, heavy duty staple used to staple together just a couple of sheets will often cause the ends of the staple to over-lap on the reverse side of the document.

Pre-packed staples are held together in ribbon-like strips and inserted into a stapler. The individual staples are held in the ribbon by an adhesive layer. In contrast, individual staples that are cut from a reel of wire will not have the adhesive and the cutting of the individual staple is done by a sharp blade. If there are any imperfections in the cutting blade, these might show up at the endings of the individual staples which would have a distinctive appear-ance that could, in principle, provide an evidential link between a staple and a stapling machine. Of course, it is still necessary to compare the physical prop-erties of the wire, such as its colour and thickness.

6.4 Adhesives

Adhesives can be used in a number of ways in a document. Pages in a pad are often held in place at one edge by a thin adhesive layer. Of course, adhesive can be applied as glue to a document or perhaps as a material from an adhesive tape. Adhesives are derived from a number of sources including natural biological products (which typically use a protein called collagen that is treated to produce glue) and hydrocarbons (which are products of the petroleum industry). Most modern adhesives fall into the latter category.

Various resins and plasticiser petroleum compounds have a tacky or sticky property that is ideal for adhesives and adhesive tapes. These compounds can be analysed using many of the techniques referred to in Chapter 7. For example:

- Gas chromatography/mass spectrometry (Aziz et al., 2008). The authors found some complex hydrocarbon compounds were used by a number of different manufacturers; but the amounts of each compound varied such that, using a statistical method, tapes from different sources could be distinguished from one another.

- Atomic force microscopy (Canetta & Adya, 2011). This method showed that the adhesive layer on pressure sensitive tapes can vary in its nano-scale (10^{-9} metre structure) and also in the amount of force exerted by the adhesive layer (its 'stickiness').

- Attenuated total reflection Fourier transform infrared spectroscopy (ATR FT-IR) (Kumooka, 2009). Infrared spectroscopy was used to obtain the spectra which were then analysed using cluster analysis to group the adhesives into similar kinds.

Using such analytical methods, it is possible to create a database of available adhesive materials against which suspect materials can be compared. The value of different techniques in their ability to discriminate between adhesives can help decide which analytical methods are most appropriate (Maynard et al., 2001).

6.5 Miscellaneous materials

(Dry transfers are described in Chapter 5 as they are akin to a form of printing and are often used to simulate printed material.)

No list of components of documents can be exhaustive as anything can crop up, from lipstick used as a writing medium to a piece of tape stuck to a document. In such circumstances, the forensic examiner will need to use their own experience and quite possibly the expertise of colleagues to assist them with such examinations. It may even be necessary to conduct some small-scale research or experiments to gain background information to enable findings to be interpreted. The reporting of conclusions in such cases needs to be based on sound methodology and properly recorded details and results so that the conclusions can be reasonably challenged by others if necessary.

6.6   Case notes relating to the physical components of a document

In all document examination cases it is a good idea to note some basic details of what is present on a document, such as the colour of inks used or the type of pen used. However, the focus on the physical components of a document is usually most important in cases where alteration to a document has been alleged (discussed in more detail in Chapter 8). In many cases a careful visual examination, possibly with microscopy or other optical (non-destructive) methods, will suffice. The important point is that the findings relating to the paper and ink, and other components where relevant, are noted, the methods of examination are described clearly and the results are recorded, ideally photographically so as to aid the demonstration of findings if oral evidence is needed at a subsequent hearing. If photographs are taken and form part of the notes, then the conditions in which they were taken (such as with transmitted light when showing a watermark) and any magnification used should also be noted.

Measurements taken must be recorded (such as the thickness of a sheet of paper) and if specialist lighting is used the conditions must be recorded (such as the wavelength of the incident light and of any filters used).

In other words, the case notes should be such that another person can read them and be able to reconstruct what was done, what was observed and what conclusions were reached with regard to the inks, paper and other components present.

6.7   Reports relating to the physical components of a document

It is unusual for a document examiner to be asked to examine paper or ink or any other component of a document in isolation. Rather it is usually in the context of allegations of alterations to a document that these aspects need to be examined (see Chapter 8).

If, for example, an examination of some paper is carried out to establish its date of production, then the report will benefit from some background explanation of relevant aspects, such as a description of paper making and any supporting witness information (such as a statement from a manager of a paper mill saying when certain papers were made and using what materials). This will enable the reader to comprehend the significance of the expert's findings and conclusions in what otherwise is likely to be unfamiliar to them from their general knowledge.

The avoidance of technical terms may be impossible in such cases, but the use of a glossary or brief explanations in brackets will assist the reader when jargon is unavoidable. As with any complex report, a brief summary describing the conclusions in the absence of explanatory findings will make it clear to the reader what the expert's opinion is.

Paper examination: a worked example

In this section an example of how to approach a case and make notes is demonstrated. The worked example is intended to show a general process in terms of thinking and doing, rather than an expectation that the reader will 'test' themselves to see if they can get the 'right' answer (although getting the 'right' answer could be regarded as a welcome bonus!).

It should be stressed that there are a number of different ways to make notes, and the intention here is to show the kinds of issues that need to be considered and how these interrelate with the observation process leading to a conclusion.

Case circumstances

A threatening note, item 1, has been pushed through the letterbox of Mr Howard. Mr Howard suspects that Mr Christie put the note through his door as they are in dispute about matters at work and there have been incidents of cars being damaged.

Mr Christie has refused handwriting samples, but a search of his home found a piece of paper, item 2, pushed down the side of his armchair.

Purpose

To compare the two pieces of paper to determine whether or not they were once part of a single sheet of paper.

Items submitted

Item 1: Threatening note (Figure 6.3)

Item 2: Piece of blank, crumpled paper (Figure 6.4)

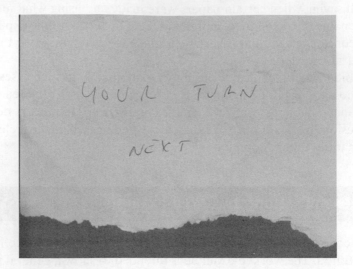

Figure 6.3   Worked example: Note item 1.

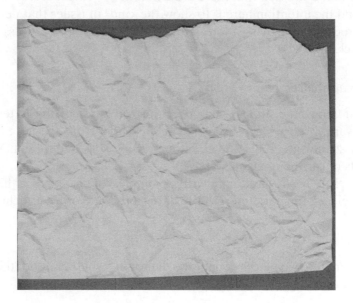

Figure 6.4   Worked example: Crumpled piece of paper item 2.

Case notes (see also Section 8.2.1)

Observations	Thoughts
<ul><li>The colour of the paper of items 1 and 2 is similar.</li><li>The appearance of items 1 and 2 under ultraviolet light is similar showing the presence of optical brighteners as expected in this kind of paper.</li><li>There is no watermark apparent in either item 1 or 2.</li><li>The dimensions of item 2 are difficult to measure accurately because it has been heavily crumpled, which will tend to make it smaller as flattening it out to its original state is impossible. However, placing the torn edges close to one another – see photograph (Figure 6.5) – it is clear that the width of the sheets is about the same.</li><li>The thickness is also difficult to measure accurately because of the crumpling, but the measurements taken from both sheets show a similar thickness.</li></ul>	Is the paper of items 1 and 2 similar?
Note that some of the areas of tearing are not clean but rather have sheared through the paper thickness – see photograph (Figure 6.6). This can cause apparent mismatches in the torn edge but can be resolved if the sheared areas coincide. Careful examination of these areas shows a very close correspondence between items 1 and 2 adding significant additional evidence.	Based on the observations so far, it is possible that items 1 and 2 were originally part of the same piece of paper. But when the two torn edges are brought close to one another, some parts of the tear appear to match better than others as shown on the photograph (Figure 6.5). Is there an explanation for this apparent anomaly?

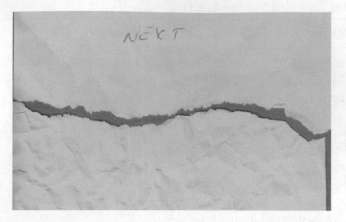

Figure 6.5 Worked example: Torn edges from items 1 and 2 in close proximity.

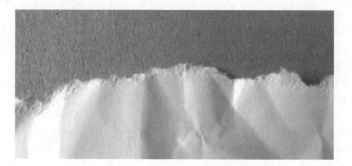

Figure 6.6 Worked example: Paper sheared.

Observations	Thoughts
If the sheared edges are laid under one another more carefully, a better physical fit between the torn edges is apparent – see photograph (Figure 6.7).	Alternatives to consider: • Items 1 and 2 from different sheets and tear similarity is a coincidence. • Items 1 and 2 from different sheets but part of a set of sheets torn together. • Items 1 and 2 are part of the same sheet.

Observations	Thoughts
	The physical fit is not perfect along the whole length of the sheet. Could this mean that items 1 and 2 were not part of the same sheet and that the similar tear patterns are a chance coincidence? The element of coincidence can definitely be rejected given the level of similarity.
	Could two or more sheets have been torn simultaneously to give similar tear patterns that might account for the overall high level of similarity but also the not quite perfect match? This too can be ruled out once the extremely close pattern match of the sheared paper surface areas is taken into account.
	There is only one appropriate conclusion, which is that there is conclusive evidence that items 1 and 2 were originally part of the same piece of paper, for which the overwhelming evidence of similarity has been described above, and that the unmatched areas are due to subsequent changes to the torn edges of item 2, in particular its treatment of being found in a crumpled state in a confined space.

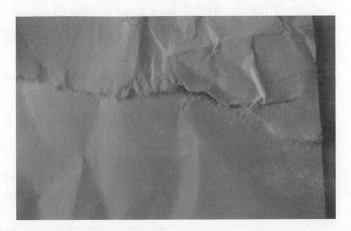

Figure 6.7   Worked example: Sheared edges overlapped to show correct physical fit.

Report of Forensic Expert

(Again, it is stressed that this report is intended to demonstrate an approach and not to be a test of getting the 'right' answer.)

Qualifications and experience ...

Scope of expertise ...

Items examined

I have examined the following items at the instruction of (the investigating authority). They were received at the laboratory on (dates).

Item 1: Threatening note

Item 2: Piece of torn paper

Purpose

I have compared items 1 and 2 with a view to determining whether or not they were originally part of the same sheet of paper.

Findings

The papers of items 1 and 2 are similar in their general characteristics such as colour and dimensions.

The torn edges of items 1 and 2 are similar in many respects in terms of their overall shape, although there are some regions that are not so well matched. However, there are some areas of the torn edges that match particularly closely in significant respects.

In my opinion, there is conclusive evidence that items 1 and 2 were originally part of the same sheet of paper, and the slight differences between them can readily be attributed to the subsequent treatment of item 2, in particular causing it to crumple and deform.

Summary

There is conclusive evidence that items 1 and 2 were originally part of the same sheet of paper.

References

Aziz, N., Greenwood, P. F., Grice, K., et al. (2008). Chemical fingerprinting of adhesive tapes by GCMS detection of petroleum hydrocarbon products. *Journal of Forensic Sciences*, 53(5), 1130–1137. doi:10.1111/j.1556-4029.2008.00798.x.

Biermann, C. J. (1996). *Handbook of Pulping and Papermaking*. London: Academic Press.

Brunelle, R. L., & Crawford, K. R. (2003). *Advances in the Forensic Analysis and Dating of Writing Ink*. Springfield, IL, USA: Charles C. Thomas.

Canetta, E., & Adya, A. K. (2011). Atomic force microscopic investigation of commercial pressure sensitive adhesives for forensic analysis. *Forensic Science International*, 210(1–3), 16–25. doi:10.1016/j.forsciint.2011.01.029.

Kumooka, Y. (2009). Hierarchical cluster analysis as a tool for preliminary discrimination of ATR-FT-IR spectra of OPP acrylic and rubber-based adhesives. *Forensic Science International*, 189(1–3), 104–110. doi:10.1016/j.forsciint.2009.04.025.

Maynard, P., Gates, K., Roux, C., & Lennard, C. (2001). Adhesive tape analysis: Establishing the evidential value of specific techniques. *Journal of Forensic Sciences*, 46(2), 280–287.

7
Analytical Techniques Used in Document Examination

In this chapter, the principles behind the main categories of analytical techniques will be described in a relatively straightforward manner with the intention that those less familiar with the chemistry involved will at least be able to understand the main ideas behind the methods. For those with more chemical knowledge, more in depth information and examples of published papers that use the techniques can be found in the Further Reading section of the Preface.

Ink, being a coloured material, is obviously amenable to a simple visual examination. For most people, colour discrimination is generally very good and this provides a useful starting point for comparing inks. However, other more objective methods are available that use the optical and chemical properties of ink. The scientific value of any technique can be compared to that of other techniques available so that the potential (evidential) gain of using a more sophisticated method can be weighed up against the probably less costly and less time-consuming simpler technique. Thus, while it may be possible to use ever more sophisticated pieces of equipment, their use needs to be justified in terms of both the likely evidential gain and the practical costs.

Chemical comparison and analysis of the materials on documents essentially involves the examination of the materials from which documents are composed, typically inks (which come to be on a document via handwritten entries, typescript and computer printers and conventional printing), toners and paper (and occasionally other materials such as adhesives may be pertinent to a case). The composition of inks and toners in particular has developed over the years and the technological instrumentation available has become increasingly sophisticated. As new analytical methods are developed, they are often applied to the examination of inks and toners, and for this reason the

Foundations of Forensic Document Analysis: Theory and Practice, First Edition. Michael Allen.
© 2016 John Wiley & Sons, Ltd. Published 2016 by John Wiley & Sons, Ltd.
Companion Website: www.wiley.com/go/allen/forensicanalysis

literature contains a wide variety of approaches to their analysis. No single method has become the standard. However, there are overall processes that can be followed, and these are described in ASTM 1422-05 and 1789-04.

An operational laboratory will not contain the whole range of equipment needed for all the various methods available. The methods used by a forensic document examiner will be constrained by the equipment either in their laboratory or to which they may be able to gain access, for example in a university department. Other constraints are: (i) the sample preparation needed, particularly if it involves removal of ink from the document since such a 'destructive' technique may not be sanctioned by the investigator as it materially changes (albeit minimally) the document, (ii) the cost of the technique and (iii) the expertise involved in using the technique and interpreting the results obtained by the experts.

Different techniques are likely to be better for particular types of ink so there is no one standard technique that is suitable for all case examinations. For this reason, it is a necessary preliminary step to identify the means by which the ink came to be on the paper (is it original pen-on-paper ink or from a scanned copy printed with a computer printer?) and this is generally determined by microscopic examination as described in the relevant previous chapters. Once this has been determined, then the techniques available to a particular laboratory can be surveyed to decide which method (or methods) is best to take the examination further.

In most situations there is no shortage of ink to examine, so if one method does not assist then it may be possible to try other methods (for example infrared spectroscopy and Raman spectroscopy could be tried and if they do not help then x-ray fluorescence could be tried (Li et al., 2014; Zięba-Palus & Kunicki, 2006). Such approaches reflect the uncertain nature of the ink and paper combination being examined and the storage conditions and the effects this will have.

In many cases, the forensic need is to *compare* samples of ink (are these two inks similar or different?) rather than to *analyse* them (what is this ink made up of?).

In forensic document examination, materials (such as ink) that might be examined using one or other of the techniques described below are often already associated with a substrate (such as a sheet of paper). Thus, ink is probably on a document (rather than still in the pen) and this raises the possibility that the ink and the paper may interact in some way that could affect the results of a chemical examination. For this reason, it is good practice to examine not only the material of interest (the ink) but also to run a 'blank' from the substrate so that any components that are from the substrate can be 'subtracted' from the result for the test substance. For example, if a blue ink was removed from a sheet of paper and when examined components A, B, C and D were present, but when the paper on its own (with no ink) was examined it contained component D, then the presence of component D in the ink sample may be due its presence in the paper rather than the ink. (Being very cautious, the coincidental possibility that component D was present in both the paper and the ink may need to be investigated if relevant.) The important point, however, is that any potential 'contamination' of the test substance by its association with another material must be taken into account when interpreting the results of the various techniques.

While there are many chemical analytical techniques available to the forensic document examiner, there a smaller number of underlying principles on which they are based. These include the *separation* of components of a mix (typical of that found in inks), the *identification of the molecules* present and the *identification of the elements* present. (See Box 7.1 for a brief description of some of the key concepts to assist readers who are less familiar with chemistry.)

The net result is an array of techniques that use different *properties* of the chemicals present in, say, a sample of ink to either compare or analyse different samples of forensic interest and a number of the methods that exploit these properties will now be described.

Box 7.1 The foundations of chemical analysis

All matter is made up of atoms. There are over 100 different kinds of atom (known as elements – such as hydrogen, carbon and oxygen) and they can be found in the periodic table, which arranges them according to certain properties that they have.

Atoms are made up of three types of particle known as protons (which carry a positive charge), neutrons (which carry no charge) and electrons (which carry a negative charge). All atoms of a given element (such as oxygen) have the same number of protons and electrons (eight of each in the case of oxygen) so that the atom is neutral (the charges cancel each other out so it carries no net charge). However, it is possible for electrons to be added to or removed from an atom which thereby produces a 'charged atom' or more precisely an *ion*.

A molecule is made up of two or more atoms joined together by a bond. Some molecules are very simple (such as molecular oxygen, which consists of two oxygen atoms linked together by a bond) whereas other molecules may be very large and complex containing many different types of atoms (compounds) in different linked configurations (for example cellulose, which forms the basis of most paper).

Chemical analysis seeks to determine what molecules or atoms (elements) are present in a test material (such as a sample of ink). The analytical techniques may be used to simply compare two or more samples to determine whether they are similar or not without necessarily trying to establish what it is that is present. The ways in which the analytical techniques achieve this differ from one technique to another and use different properties of the molecules of the test material (such as their ability to form ions or the ways in which their bonds respond to light). In other words, the differing properties of the test materials, which are caused by the underlying physics of the chemicals present, are exploited by the various analytical techniques.

7.1   Chromatography

The purpose of chromatography is to *separate* mixtures of components in a test material (such as ink). In some cases this separation may be sufficient, for example when *comparing* two or more materials to see if they do or do not contain the same mix of components. However, as each separate component is isolated by the chromatographic process, there is the possibility to then *analyse* each separated component to determine what it is.

The test material is separated by moving it in a mobile phase (liquid or gas) through a stationary phase. Components with a high affinity for the stationary phase move more slowly through the column, while those with a lower affinity emerge from the column earlier. A number of stationary phases can be used, but examples are alumina or silica materials, which have the appearance of a white powder-like substance. In practice, the components of a test mixture are dissolved into a solvent (the mobile phase) and the different components are separated according to how they interact with the material in the structure which forms the stationary phase that is present in the experimental set up. (The nature of the interaction is complex and can vary according to many different factors. In general, experience has shown that certain combinations of stationary phase, mobile phase and experimental conditions – such as temperature – are optimal for different types of chemical being tested.)

There are variations of this general separation process that broadly fall into three categories:

- thin layer chromatography, in which the stationary phase is a thin layer of material supported, for example, on a glass or aluminium plate;

- liquid chromatography, in which the solution containing the mixture is forced through a thin column packed with a stationary phase material; and

- gas chromatography where the test mixture is in gaseous form and passes through a narrow column the surface of which is coated with a stationary phase material.

Once the chemicals have been separated, there has to be a way of detecting them. With thin layer chromatography of inks, for example, the coloured components are visible to the naked eye. But if a chemical is not coloured, then other means of detecting it must be used. There are a number of such detectors that depend on the properties of the chemicals being analysed. The mechanisms by which detectors work are complex and not relevant here, but the output from the detector is related to the amount of material being detected (analogous to how intense a coloured spot is on a TLC plate to the naked eye). This means that the output from a detector is quantitative. The quantitative data then provide a means to form a database of *known chemicals* and their chromatographic properties against which the test material can be compared, hence suggesting the identity of the test chemicals present.

Confirmation of the identity of chemicals present can be achieved in a number of ways. For example, the output from the gas chromatography column can be analysed using other methods, typically mass spectrometry (see Section 7.2 below). This double approach is one that is widely practised in forensic chemistry as it is unlikely that two chemicals will behave similarly when analysed using two different analytical methods. In other words, inadvertently mis-identifying a chemical becomes less likely the more techniques that are used to analyse it, and in practice two techniques (such as chromatography and mass spectrometry) are normally sufficient to provide reliable identification.

7.1.1 Thin layer chromatography (TLC)

When used to examine ink present on a document, TLC is a destructive method as it requires a sample of ink to be removed. The sample size needed is small, however, and providing appropriate permission is obtained to take a sample, the slight damage to the document is not usually likely to cause any subsequent (legal) difficulty regarding the 'completeness' of the document. TLC is also relatively cheap to perform and, although it does require careful practice to perfect, it is a fairly straightforward technique to use.

In thin layer chromatography, a sample of ink is removed from the document or taken directly from a pen using a solvent. A small spot of the ink sample is placed close to one edge of a chromatography 'plate' (typically a layer of powder-like silica gel on a glass support). The plate is then placed into a shallow bath containing another solvent (the mobile phase), which moves up the plate (the stationary phase) by capillary action and as it does so separates the components in the ink samples which can then be compared one with another.

However, interpreting the results using TLC requires some caution. As noted above, it is always necessary to run a paper 'blank' and care needs to be taken as it is possible for documents to be accidentally contaminated with inks from, for example, other pages which come into contact with it, not least because ink is a liquid material when placed on the paper and it may take days or weeks to fully dry. Further, while ink formulas do vary from one manufacturer to another, there are likely to be similarities in ink composition between manufacturers since certain dyes and pigments are widely used (added to which there is the possibility that an *ink* manufacturer could supply their product to more than one *pen* manufacturer). Because of such factors, it is generally possible to show *differences* between inks by the different separated components present. However, if two samples show similar patterns of separated components this may simply be a reflection of the wide availability of some ranges of pens in the marketplace rather than providing significant evidence that the same pen/ink was used.

Assessing the separated components on a plate can be done visually, perhaps using other light sources such as ultraviolet light to illuminate the plate. This obviously is a non-quantitative approach, although some approximation of the amount of a separated component may be possible depending on the *intensity* of the spot on the TLC plate (a faint spot indicating that not much of the component is present, a darker spot indicating more is present). However, there are methods to measure the amounts of material present for each separated component, such as densitometry (which measures optical density of material present) or by using image analysis software. The position of the separated component is usually measured in relation to the position that the mobile phase reached – referred to as the R_f value. Hence two components of an ink that have similar *colour* but which have different R_f *values* are in fact different chemicals. A typical plate is shown in Figure 7.1.

Published articles that have used TLC to examine inks include:

- Roux et al. (1999), in which the usefulness of TLC is compared to optical methods of examining ink;

- Djozan et al., (2008), which uses image analysis software to interpret the separated spots on the plate;

- Neumann and Margot (2009a,b,c), which are a series of papers that focus primarily on TLC of ink and how the evidence should be handled to achieve reliable results.

7.1.2 High performance liquid chromatography (HPLC)

In HPLC, the two-dimensional plate that is used in TLC is replaced by a tubular column (typically about 3 mm in diameter and up to about 25 cm in length) that is packed with a stationary phase material, such as silica or various polymers. The ink to be examined is forced through the column in a solvent under pressure. Separation of components of the ink again depends on their interaction with the stationary phase, with different components coming out of the column at different (retention) times. There are various

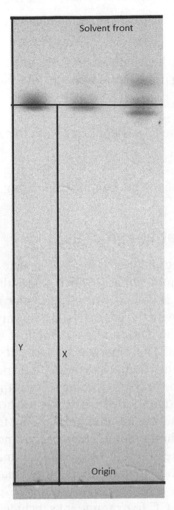

Figure 7.1 A typical thin line chromatography plate showing the separation of ink components. Each component has its own separation factor, known as R_f, which is calculated by dividing the distance the component has migrated (X) by the distance travelled by the solvent (Y). *(See insert for colour representation of the figure.)*

parameters that can be changed with this technique, such as the solvent used, the pressure applied and the particle size of the stationary phase, all of which can affect the results obtained.

While TLC produced a physical record of the separation of the components in ink on the plate, HPLC produces a stream of solvent from the far end of the column and the presence of material in the solvent has to be *detected* by some means. One such is a UV detector, which responds to changes in the ultraviolet response of the material as it emerges from the column. The extent of the detector response is related to the amount of material being detected and so provides a quantitative result.

Papers that have used HPLC to examine inks include:

- Kher et al. (2006) in which ballpen inks are analysed and the results statistically processed using principal component analysis and linear discriminant analysis;

- Wang et al. (2008) used a variant known as ion pairing HPLC to compare fountain pen inks;

- Liu et al. (2006) classified gel pen inks also using ion pair HPLC.

7.1.3   Gas chromatography (GC)

In GC, the material being analysed is heated to make it a gas and this is mixed with a carrier gas (the mobile phase) which passes the sample through a thin tube, or column, which is coated with a particular material (the stationary phase) that can interact with the gas material being analysed thereby affecting its passage along the tube. Different gases interact with different stationary phases in complex ways. The emergence of the test gas from the column (having passed through the column assisted by a carrier gas, such as hydrogen, in a manner similar to the pressure forcing solvent through a HPLC column) is detected (there are a number of detection methods) and the time taken reflects the interaction between the material being tested and the stationary phase coated on the column. Some chemicals do not readily form gases at the required temperatures used in GC, and such materials may need to be chemically pre-treated so as to make them more volatile (a process known as derivatisation).

Papers that have used GC to examine inks include:

- Bugler et al. (2005) used GC-MS to analyse the non-coloured components of ballpen ink;

- Li et al. (2014) examined gel pen inks.

GC is widely used with mass spectrometry (see Section 7.2).

7.2   Mass spectrometry (MS)

Mass spectrometry works by ionising compounds to generate charged molecules and molecule fragments and measuring the mass to charge ratio. The sample to be analysed is typically bombarded with electrons, which may cause molecules to ionise and to break up into fragments. The charged fragments and molecules are then subjected to a magnetic field that separates them according to how much charge and mass they have. The output requires the detection of the charged particles and the results are compared against a database of known substances to identify the components in the test material. Mass spectrometry generally requires the substance being analysed to be volatile (so that it can enter the gas phase relatively easily). Recent developments such as electrospray mass spectrometry mean that even molecules of low volatility can be analysed by mass spectrometry.

Papers that have used MS to examine inks include:

- Williams et al. (2009), in which electrospray ionisation was used to examine ballpen, gel pen and rollerball inks;

- Coumbaros et al. (2009) used a variant of MS known as time of flight secondary ion mass spectrometry (TOF-SIMS) to examine ballpen inks;

- Gallidabino et al. (2011) and Weyermann et al. (2012) used the same variant of MS to examine ballpen inks and gel pen inks respectively.

- Houlgrave et al. (2013) used another variant of MS known as AccuTOF DART (Direct Analysis in Real Time) Mass Spectrometry to analyse components of inkjet inks.

7.3 Spectroscopy

Spectroscopy uses the fact that chemicals (such as those present in inks, for example) can interact with visible light or light of other wavelengths (see also Box 8.1). The wavelength absorbed depends on the atoms and the bonds present between them in the molecules being analysed (see Box 7.1).

In practice, the result of a spectroscopic analysis is a spectrum showing peaks and troughs at different wavelengths, and this can be compared to the spectrum from other samples.

Comparing inks by their response to visible, infrared and ultraviolet light is a standard technique in document examination and the results can be recorded using suitable cameras. Various pieces of equipment have been devised, aimed at document examination, that exploit these properties and are also very valuable when looking at some of the optical devices found in security documents (see also Chapter 5). The use of such equipment would be routine following a visual and/or microscopic examination of the document when assessing it for evidence of alteration (see Chapter 8).

7.3.1 Infrared spectroscopy

The bonds that link the atoms together in the chemicals being analysed can vibrate in a variety of ways, such as symmetrical and asymmetrical vibrations, rocking and twisting. The nature of the vibrations that occur will determine the infrared absorption spectrum for that substance.

In practice, a beam of light is shone onto the sample, and when the frequency is the same as that of a vibrational energy in the sample, the frequency is absorbed. This can be measured and is indicative of the material present.

Papers that have used infrared spectroscopy to examine inks include:

- Dirwono et al. (2010) used a variant known as Fourier transform infrared spectroscopy (FTIR) to examine the red inks of seals that are commonly used in some east Asian countries instead of a signature.

- Almeida Assis et al. (2012) analysed black toner with diamond cell FTIR,

- Sonnex et al. (2014) used infrared spectroscopy to help identify forged currency.

7.3.2 Raman spectroscopy

If the light shone onto the sample is of a single wavelength (monochromatic light typically from a laser beam), then the scattering of that light is dependent on the vibration of the molecules present. This is the principle behind Raman spectroscopy. The information obtained is similar to infrared spectroscopy but, because of the difference in the methods, it yields additional information about the test chemicals. The technique is non-destructive (assuming a low power laser is used) and non-invasive and is thus an ideal method of forensic analysis.

One problem that can occur in Raman spectroscopy is fluorescence caused by the laser. Even though the fluorescence is relatively weak it is much stronger than the Raman scattering and saturates the detector, which is designed for very low intensity light levels. One way to overcome this problem is to treat a small portion of the ink with a gold or silver colloid. This quenches the fluorescence and provides a greatly enhanced Raman spectrum (over a million times increases in sensitivity have been claimed) of the fluorescent material. This variant is known as Surface Enhanced Resonance Raman Spectroscopy (SERRS).

Papers that have used Raman spectroscopy to examine inks include:

- Seifar et al. (2001) and White (2003) in which SERRS is used to examine ballpen inks;

- Raza & Saha (2013) used Raman spectroscopy to analyse stamp pad inks;

- Braz et al. (2013) analysed inks using normal Raman and also surface enhanced Raman spectroscopy;

- Bell et al. (2013) compared liquid and gel inks using standard Raman, SERRS and other established methods to see which were most suitable.

7.3.3   UV-visible (UV-vis) spectroscopy

When light of the correct wavelength is shone at molecules, the electrons in the chemical bonds can absorb energy. Dyes and pigments are commonly found in inks and these molecules absorb light in the visible region of the electromagnetic spectrum. Thus a red ink will absorb light from all but the red part of the spectrum. The red light is reflected and perceived by the eye as red. The absorption of light plotted against wavelength is the so-called electronic spectrum (so called because it is the electrons that are responsible for the absorption). The absorption of the light often extends into the ultraviolet region of the spectrum, and hence the technique is often referred to as UV-vis spectroscopy. Generally, recording the UV-vis spectrum requires the ink to be in solution and thus it has to be removed from the page. More recently, instruments have been developed to measure the spectrum in situ, thus requiring no destructive pre-treatment.

Papers that have used UV-vis spectroscopy to examine documents include:

- Adam et al. (2008) in which the results obtained from UV-visible absorption spectroscopy of ballpen inks were analysed using a statistical method known as principal components analysis;

- Causin et al. (2012) used a variant called diffuse-reflectance ultraviolet-visible-near infrared spectrophotometry to distinguish between sheets of paper that were visually similar.

7.4   X-ray fluorescence (XRF)

XRF is based on the fact that when substances are exposed to x-rays (which have a short wavelength and a high energy) they cause electrons to be lost from the atoms present and this creates an unstable ion (see Box 7.1). The lost electron(s) create spaces in the atomic structure of the atom into which other electrons fall to fill in the gap and this leads to the *emission* of further energetic x-rays, the wavelengths of which are characteristic for different atoms. In this way the identity of the elements present in a test material can be determined by comparing the results against a database of results from known elements – so-called elemental analysis.

Papers that have used XRF to examine inks include:

- Zięba-Palus & Kunicki (2006) used XRF, infrared absorption and Raman spectroscopy in the analysis of ballpen and gel pen inks;

- Chu et al. (2013) used XRF to compare laser toners;

- Trzcinska (2006) used FTIR to classify toners and then XRF to gain further discrimination between toners.

7.5   Electrophoresis

Different components of a mixture are separated in an electric field that is applied through a gel-like medium. Tiny samples are placed onto the gel and an electric field is applied, which has a different effect on different compounds present. The movement of the components is, therefore, determined by the electrical and physical properties of the chemicals being analysed.

Papers that have used electrophoresis to examine inks include:

- Szafarska et al. (2011) used electrophoresis to compare inkjet inks;

- Krol et al. (2013) used two variants of electrophoresis to study stamp inks, the variations being in both the electrophoretic process itself and the type of detector used.

7.6   Case notes when scientific equipment is used

The use of equipment must of course be recorded in the case notes. If more than one similar piece of equipment is available, then it is important that the particular machine used is noted (for example, gas chromatography machine number 1 – rather than number 2 – was used). The reason that it is important to record this information is that if at some point the particular piece of equipment is checked and found not to have been working properly, then it may be necessary to repeat the relevant analyses. Of course, it is a requirement that all pieces of equipment are regularly checked and any relevant information should be available to show that the equipment is working properly.

The details that need recording will depend to some extent on the equipment used and the particular circumstances of the case. However, as also noted at the end of Chapter 6, the case notes should contain all relevant information regarding methods used, equipment used, the conditions (such as the type of column used in gas chromatography) and any other relevant details that would allow another person to recreate what was done and come up with the same results.

Some equipment produces large amounts of data and associated paper plots. These of course also form part of the case notes. Much data is also capable of being stored in a computer, be it digital photographs showing inks under specialist lighting conditions or peaks of different elements present in a sample of paper. Electronic records must also be linked in some way to the physical case file containing all other paperwork relating to the case. Indeed, there is a gradual trend away from paper-based records to electronic records but this is far from complete and much information is still stored in traditional filing cabinets.

7.7 Reports in cases where scientific equipment is used

The use of specialist equipment is almost always in the context of some aspect of a case, such as alterations to a document. Where the findings of an expert required the use of equipment, that use needs to be included in the report. The *reason* for needing to use the equipment usually suffices (as opposed to an explanation of how the equipment works). For example, if thin layer chromatography of ink is carried out, the reason for so doing could be that the inks could not be differentiated visually using specialist lighting so chemical analysis was done. When it is necessary to refer to the technical details of the equipment or its use, non-technical wordings are ideal, but if they cannot be avoided a short explanation as to their meaning will assist the non-expert reader.

Worked example

In view of the nature of the information in this chapter there is no worked example.

References

Adam, C. D., Sherratt, S. L., & Zholobenko, V. L. (2008). Classification and individualisation of black ballpoint pen inks using principal component analysis of UV–vis absorption spectra. *Forensic Science International*, 174(1), 16–25. doi: 10.1016/j.forsciint.2007.02.029.

Almeida Assis, A. C., Barbosa, M. F., et al. (2012). Diamond cell Fourier transform infrared spectroscopy transmittance analysis of black toners on questioned documents. *Forensic Science International*, 214(1–3), 59–66. doi:10.1016/j.forsciint.2011.07.019.

Bell, S. E. J., Stewart, S. P., Ho, Y. C., et al. (2013). Comparison of the discriminating power of raman and surface-enhanced raman spectroscopy with established techniques for the examination of liquid and gel inks. *Journal of Raman Spectroscopy*, 44(4), 509–517. doi:10.1002/jrs.4202.

Braz, A., Lopez-Lopez, M., & Garcia-Ruiz, C. (2013). Raman spectroscopy for forensic analysis of inks in questioned documents. *Forensic Science International*, 232(1–3), 206–212. doi:10.1016/j.forsciint.2013.07.017.

Bugler, J. H., Buchner, H., & Dallmayer, A. (2005). Characterization of ballpoint pen inks by thermal desorption and gas chromatography-mass spectrometry. *Journal of Forensic Sciences*, 50(5), 1209–1214.

Causin, V., Casamassima, R., Marruncheddu, G., et al. (2012). The discrimination potential of diffuse-reflectance ultraviolet-visible-near infrared spectrophotometry for the forensic analysis of paper. *Forensic Science International*, 216(1–3), 163–167. doi:10.1016/j.forsciint.2011.09.015.

Chu, P., Cai, B. Y., Tsoi, Y. K., et al. (2013). Forensic analysis of laser printed ink by X-ray fluorescence and laser-excited plume fluorescence. *Analytical Chemistry*, 85(9), 4311–4315. doi:10.1021/ac400318q.

Coumbaros, J., Kirkbride, K. P., Klass, G., & Skinner, W. (2009). Application of time of flight secondary ion mass spectrometry to the in situ analysis of ballpoint pen inks on paper. *Forensic Science International*, 193(1–3), 42–46. doi: 10.1016/j.forsciint.2009.08.020.

Dirwono, W., Park, J. S., Agustin-Camacho, M., et al. (2010). Application of micro-attenuated total reflectance FTIR spectroscopy in the forensic study of questioned documents involving red seal inks. *Forensic Science International*, 199(1–3), 6–8.

Djozan, D., Baheri, T., Karimian, G., & Shahidi, M. (2008). Forensic discrimination of blue ballpoint pen inks based on thin layer chromatography and image analysis. *Forensic Science International*, 179(2–3), 199–205. doi:10.1016/j.forsciint.2008.05.013 ER.

Gallidabino, M., Weyermann, C., & Marquis, R. (2011). Differentiation of blue ballpoint pen inks by positive and negative mode LDI-MS. *Forensic Science International*, 204(1–3), 169–178. doi:10.1016/j.forsciint.2010.05.027.

Houlgrave, S., LaPorte, G. M., Stephens, J. C., & Wilson, J. L. (2013). The classification of inkjet inks using AccuTOF DART (direct analysis in real time) mass SpectrometryA preliminary study. *Journal of Forensic Sciences*, 58(3), 813–821. doi:10.1111/1556-4029.12048.

Kher, A., Mulholland, M., Green, E., & Reedy, B. (2006). Forensic classification of ballpoint pen inks using high performance liquid chromatography and infrared spectroscopy with principal components analysis and linear discriminant analysis. *Vibrational Spectroscopy*, 40(2), 270–277. doi:10.1016/j.vibspec.2005.11.002.

Krol, M., Kula, A., & Koscielniak, P. (2013). Application of MECC-DAD and CZE-MS to examination of color stamp inks for forensic purposes. *Forensic Science International*, 233(1–3), 140–148. doi:10.1016/j.forsciint.2013.09.006.

Li, B., Xie, P., Guo, Y., & Fei, Q. (2014). GC analysis of black gel pen ink stored under different conditions. *Journal of Forensic Sciences*, 59(2), 543–549. doi:10.1111/1556-4029.12313.

Liu, Y., Yu, J., Xie, M., et al. (2006). Classification and dating of black gel pen ink by ion-pairing high-performance liquid chromatography. *Journal of Chromatography A*, 1135(1), 57–64. doi:10.1016/j.chroma.2006.09.031.

Neumann, C., & Margot, P. (2009a). New perspectives in the use of ink evidence in forensic science part II. development and testing of mathematical algorithms for the automatic comparison of ink samples analysed by HPTLC. *Forensic Science International*, 185(1–3), 38–50. doi:10.1016/j.forsciint.2008.12.008.

Neumann, C., & Margot, P. (2009b). New perspectives in the use of ink evidence in forensic science part III: Operational applications and evaluation. *Forensic Science International*, 192(1–3), 29–42. doi:10.1016/j.forsciint.2009.07.013.

Neumann, C., & Margot, P. (2009c). New perspectives in the use of ink evidence in forensic science: Part I. development of a quality assurance process for forensic ink analysis by HPTLC. *Forensic Science International*, 185(1–3), 29–37. doi:10.1016/j.forsciint.2008.11.016.

Raza, A., & Saha, B. (2013). Application of raman spectroscopy in forensic investigation of questioned documents involving stamp inks. *Science & Justice*, 53(3), 332–338. doi:10.1016/j.scijus.2012.11.001.

Roux, C., Novotny, M., Evans, I., & Lennard, C. (1999). A study to investigate the evidential value of blue and black ballpoint pen inks in Australia. *Forensic Science International*, 101(3), 167–176.

Seifar, R. M., Verheul, J. M., Ariese, F., et al. (2001). Applicability of surface-enhanced resonance raman scattering for the direct discrimination of ballpoint pen inks. *Analyst*, 126(8), 1418–1422. doi:10.1039/b103042f.

Sonnex, E., Almond, M. J., Baum, J. V., & Bond, J. W. (2014). Identification of forged Bank of England 20 pound banknotes using IR spectroscopy. *Spectrochimica Acta Part A-Molecular and Biomolecular Spectroscopy*, 118, 1158–1163. doi:10.1016/j.saa.2013.09.115.

Szafarska, M., Wietecha-Posluszny, R., Wozniakiewicz, M., & Koscielniak, P. (2011). Application of capillary electrophoresis to examination of color inkjet printing inks for forensic purposes. *Forensic Science International*, 212(1–3), 78–85. doi:10.1016/j.forsciint.2011.05.017.

Trzcinska, B. M. (2006). Classification of black powder toners on the basis of integrated analytical information provided by Fourier transform infrared spectrometry and X-ray fluorescence spectrometry. *Journal of Forensic Sciences*, 51(4), 919–924. doi:10.1111/j.1556-4029.2006.00167.x.

Wang, X., Yu, J., Xie, M., et al. (2008). Identification and dating of the fountain pen ink entries on documents by ion-pairing high-performance liquid chromatography. *Forensic Science International*, 180(1), 43–49. doi:10.1016/j.forsciint.2008.06.008.

Weyermann, C., Bucher, L., Majcherczyk, P., et al. (2012). Statistical discrimination of black gel pen inks analysed by laser desorption/ionization mass spectrometry. *Forensic Science International*, 217(1–3), 127–133. doi:10.1016/j.forsciint.2011.10.040.

White, P. C. (2003). In situ surface enhanced resonance raman scattering (SERRS) spectroscopy of biro inks - long term stability of colloid treated samples. *Science & Justice*, 43(3), 149–152. doi:10.1016/S1355-0306(03)71762-6.

Williams, M. R., Moody, C., Arceneaux, L., et al. (2009). Analysis of black writing ink by electrospray ionization mass spectrometry. *Forensic Science International*, 191(1–3), 97–103. doi:DOI: 10.1016/j.forsciint.2009.07.003.

Zięba-Palus, J., & Kunicki, M. (2006). Application of the micro-FTIR spectroscopy, raman spectroscopy and XRF method examination of inks. *Forensic Science International*, 158(2–3), 164–172. doi: 10.1016/j.forsciint.2005.04.044.

8
Altered and Tampered Documents

In Chapter 6, the physical materials from which documents are composed were described. Chemical methods of comparing and analysing these materials were highlighted in Chapter 7. The purpose of the current chapter is to put together this knowledge in the context of examining cases in which documents have been altered by some means. Given the variety of ways in which a document can be constructed, it is inevitable that alteration can occur in many different contexts and for a variety of reasons. An entry in a diary may need to be obliterated, the payee, date or amount on a cheque altered, or the details in a passport changed. The tools available to the document examiner are essentially the same whatever the case situation or document type, and they require the expert to have knowledge about the ways that alterations are made and the equipment and capability to reveal such changes.

In order to examine cases of alleged alteration to official documents (such as passports), the expert must have a wide-ranging knowledge of how various documents are produced and then, based on that knowledge, determine whether the suspect document has had details changed. In other document types, such as entries in a diary, the emphasis is often on a comparison between entries, particularly the inks used. But other kinds of alterations may be of interest, such as changes to a typed document, substituting one page for another in a multi-page document, or deciphering erased or obliterated entries.

There is, therefore, no such thing as a typical altered document case, so each must be treated on its own merits and the examination methods used will be those that the expert considers most appropriate in the given case.

Foundations of Forensic Document Analysis: Theory and Practice, First Edition. Michael Allen.
© 2016 John Wiley & Sons, Ltd. Published 2016 by John Wiley & Sons, Ltd.
Companion Website: www.wiley.com/go/allen/forensicanalysis

8.1   Alterations involving the examination of inks

(ASTM E1422-05 describes some of the procedures for comparing inks.)

The comparison of inks, usually from pens but also printing inks, is one of the most commonly encountered issues where alteration is alleged, particularly where the change involves adding information to an existing document. When a document is originally created it is obviously done with the materials available at that time. If at some subsequent time additions are made to that document using different materials, then the person making the alteration will desire to minimise any apparent differences in ink colour and appearance to make detection of the deed less likely.

Inks, and the pens that use them, are generally widely available and manufacturers usually make very large numbers of pens containing similar ink from a big batch. This has important consequences for the document examiner, since it means that *similarity* between inks on a document may have relatively little significance if the ink is widely available, but *differences* between inks on a document are more likely to be of forensic relevance. For this reason, it is sometimes more appropriate to conclude that various ink-written entries either can or cannot be distinguished using the methods available.

Many techniques have been applied to the forensic examination of inks, ranging from the most basic (visual examination and light microscopy) to complex and expensive equipment that may not be routinely available in many forensic laboratories (see also Chapter 7). Because inks are made up of a variety of different components, some of the techniques work better for some kinds of inks whereas other techniques work better on other inks. For these reasons, the forensic document examiner needs to apply a number of principles when deciding which approach to use in a given case. Often, the overriding factor is that the technique used should be non-destructive, that is a method that does not require removal of ink from the document. (If a destructive technique is considered, permission must be sought for any removal of ink from the document and the document photographed, or copied in some other acceptable way, so as to record its appearance before the ink is removed.) Document examiners will be limited also by the availability of equipment in their laboratory unless they have access to other equipment at, for example, a university research department. This will affect both the cost and the time required to use a particular piece of equipment, and the likelihood of obtaining a useful result must also be factored in when deciding which method(s) to use.

As a consequence of these practical limitations, some techniques are much more widely used than others. The main focus here will be on the most widely used methods of ink comparison, but some of the less frequently used techniques will also be mentioned to show the range of approaches available.

8.1.1 Microscopy of ink lines

The first and simplest technique for comparing inks is low power light microscopy. Using this, it is often possible to determine the kind of pen from which the ink came. Pen inks are either water-based or oil-based. Water-based inks are used in fountain pens and fibre-tipped pens, for example. Oil-based inks are used in ballpoint pens, which are the most frequently encountered type of pens in casework. The interaction between a water-based ink and the surface of a piece of paper differs from that between an oil-based ink and paper. This is because the paper surface is fibrous and absorbent and the more fluid water-based ink will tend to run along the fibres on the paper surface (so-called feathering) whereas oil-based inks do not do this. Oil-based inks often appear to sit on the paper surface and have a sheen to them, whereas water-based inks have more of a matt (non-shiny) appearance (see Figure 2.6).

Looking at the ink line features can, therefore, help in assessing what kind of pen was used to produce a particular ink line. Of course, the colour of the ink line is also an important property and good colour vision is an asset to the document examiner. When comparing ink lines, it should be borne in mind that the amount of ink deposited on the paper will tend to make the ink appear darker or lighter, whereas in fact the increased amount of ink may be a reflection of the pressure (greater pressure leading to more ink being deposited) or speed of writing (faster writing tending to deposit less ink on the paper surface).

The degree of colour difference will dictate whether there is a necessity to use other techniques. At an extreme, there would be no need to 'confirm' that a red ink and a blue ink are different. But if one ink appears blue/grey and the other appears blue/purple then it may be helpful to have an instrumental result to confirm and show the difference independently of the human eye.

8.1.2 Optical properties of ink

The complex mix of chemicals that make up pen inks (see Chapter 6) gives them a variety of optical properties that can be used to differentiate between them. There are a number of instruments on the market that are able to exploit this and they consist essentially of a number of different light sources to illuminate the ink (incident light), sensitive video cameras to register the light from the ink, and filters to vary both the wavelength of the light incident on the ink and the wavelengths detected from the document (see also Box 8.1).

Box 8.1 Light

The light that humans can see is usually called visible light, and it can be broken up into the colours of the rainbow (typically red, orange, yellow, green, blue, indigo and violet – although in fact the colours merge from one to the other gradually so the separation into seven colours is arbitrary). Light is often described in terms of its wave-like properties and light of different colours has different wavelengths that are typically measured in nanometres (1 nm is one billionth of a metre or 10^{-9}m). Violet light at one end of the rainbow has a shorter wavelength (about 400 nm) than red light (about 700 nm) at the other extreme.

Visible light is one (tiny) part of a much larger range of waves that includes ultraviolet light, which has a shorter wavelength than violet light, and infrared light, which has a longer wavelength than red light – both of which are invisible to humans (Figure 8.1). Other waves (such as radio waves and gamma rays) exist beyond the infrared and ultraviolet, but they are not of relevance in the examination of ink.

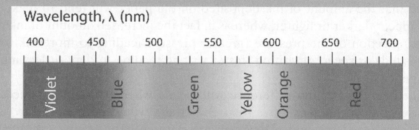

Figure 8.1   The electromagnetic spectrum. *(See insert for colour representation of the figure.)*

When light waves hit an ink line a number of things can happen. The light can be reflected back. Some of the light may be 'lost' (absorbed) by the ink. Some of the light may be absorbed by the ink which then re-emits the light at a different (longer) wavelength to that of the incident light (a process known as luminescence). The interactions between light of different wavelengths incident upon an ink line and the effect this has on the light coming from the ink line will depend upon the properties of the ink.

Viewing a document under different lighting conditions is non-destructive as it does not require the removal of ink from the document. There are different sources of illumination and filters that can be used and the expert may need to try various combinations to see which, if any, are able to distinguish between the inks of interest. Some devices are able to automatically try out the combinations and assess which seems to distinguish best between them. As noted above, however, relying on a machine to interpret the meaning of any evidence is not the purpose of the automation, which is rather to provide the expert with a possible set of parameters to look at more closely. Interpretation may need to factor in differences in pen pressure, writing speed, the effect of the background paper, or the ways in which the relevant documents have been stored.

8.1.3 Chemical analysis of inks

Many methods exist that can be used to chemically analyse inks. Some of the basic approaches are described in Chapter 7. These are continually being modified and updated as technology improves and the methods are often applied to ink comparison. However, it must be said that the majority of these methods require specialist equipment (often unavailable to the expert) and specialist knowledge to operate it and interpret the results obtained from it.

Because of its relative simplicity and low cost as a technique, thin layer chromatography is probably the most commonly used chemical method in casework, but other techniques, especially those that are non-destructive, may become increasingly widely used.

8.1.4 Where two inks intersect

See Section 10.6 in Chapter 10.

8.2 The examination of paper

(ASTM E2288-09 describes some of the procedures for comparing paper.)
Given the different fibre sources and the many treatments that paper can have, there is quite a lot of scope, in principle, to compare and analyse sheets of paper. Starting with the simplest (and cheapest) examinations, the paper's colour can be compared both under day light and under ultraviolet light. Even with this simple assessment, some care is needed as paper can vary across a batch depending on the circumstances of its manufacture (Green, 2012). The qualitative assessment of fluorescence attributable to the presence of optical brighteners can be quantified using UV-vis spectrophometry (see Chapter 7). Some care is needed when interpreting findings as small within-sheet variation can occur (Causin et al., 2012).

The optical properties of paper can be examined using transmitted light to compare the distribution of the paper fibres within the sheet (sometimes called the 'look-through') based on the potential for papers made on different machines with different starting materials to have differences in the fibre distribution within the sheet. This property of paper can also be made more objective by a mathematical analysis of the transmitted light (Berger, 2009).

If a watermark is present, this can be compared, since the design of the watermark can vary over time as the manufacturer either completely redesigns it or else uses a different version when paper production moves from one place to another. This latter situation was the basis for successfully dating a piece of paper based on the design of a watermark (Allen & Rimmer, 1988).

Of course, if the paper has been printed on, for example with margins and lines for writing, these too can be compared – although strictly they are not properties of the paper itself. The thickness of a sheet of paper can be measured using a micrometer. Typically, ten measurements are taken from different places on the sheet and averaged since the thickness can vary by a small amount across the sheet.

The various additives used in paper making can be analysed using some of the methods described in Chapter 7, but this is extremely unlikely to be needed since such methods are mostly destructive and fall into the category of 'just one more (possibly expensive) test to try to distinguish the pieces of paper' that may be hard to justify on the grounds of cost or likely outcome.

Occasionally, it is necessary to carry out an examination to determine the nature of the paper fibres themselves. This could be the case if the source or age of the paper is of particular significance to an enquiry. In order to determine the types of fibre present, a tiny (less than one square millimetre) sample of paper is removed and placed on a glass microscope slide and the fibres teased apart in water using some fine-pointed instrument. As many isolated fibres as possible need to be released from the paper, and when this process is complete the water can be dried off prior to adding a suitable dye to the sample to highlight the paper fibres' structure. Fibres from different sources have different microscopic cellular structures. Identifying the types of plant from which the fibres originate requires botanical knowledge and an atlas of photomicrographs showing fibres from the many different species of plants, although some general features may indicate the type of fibre present – for example hardwood as opposed to softwood (Biermann, 1996). This approach has been used to date the production of a piece of paper when used in conjunction with manufacturing records (Totty, Rimmer, & Steadman, 1987).

8.2.1   Torn or shredded paper

When paper is torn or cut this leads to another examination type. Tearing is by its very nature a unique event for a given sheet of paper, although if several sheets are torn together there may be some similarity in the tear patterns. Reconstructing torn sheets is generally a case of physically matching torn edges and there is rarely any difficulty with this, except if the torn pieces have been damaged or changed afterwards by, for example, the pieces being screwed up and put in a pocket for a period of time thus damaging their shape and their edges. Care may be needed to match up the fine detail of the torn edges and this can most simply and effectively be achieved by bringing the edges close together and showing that they correspond closely and taking a photograph as evidence of this (see for example Figure 6.5).

A special case of torn document is where it is torn along pre-existing perforations (see also Section 8.2.3). If, for example, the document concerned is a book of tickets from which the main piece is removed leaving a stub behind, it may well be necessary to require microscopic examination of the edges of the stubs in the book to determine which was originally attached to the ticket in question.

Shredded documents can also be reconstructed given time and patience. The ease with which this can be achieved depends on a number of factors. Obviously, the more shredded material there is the more shredded pieces from a given sheet may be muddled up with others, and for this reason if paper from a shredder is seized it is helpful to not disrupt the material so as to minimise mixing. The distinctiveness of the document is important based, for example, on the colour of the paper, the presence of printed material (such as a letterhead) or any other characteristic that helps the document examiner sort out the relevant from the irrelevant shredded strips of paper. Some shredders cross-cut the strips, producing even smaller pieces, and this makes reconstruction even harder and more time consuming. Ultimately, the effort required to reconstruct shredded documents may be justifiable if the end product is achieved since it may well be that the documentary proof it affords curtails an investigation.

8.2.2 Marks in paper

Documents that consist of a number of pages that have been joined together at some point may be taken apart and reconstituted, possibly with one or more pages added or substituted. The examination of such cases requires careful examination of all aspects of the document, including the type of paper and the handwriting or typing/printing present. In addition, the methods of joining using staples or even paperclips may provide useful evidence.

Staples on documents are often removed, leaving behind staple holes. The distance of these holes from one another will indicate the size of the staple that originally was present, although staples can move around and enlarge the holes so caution is necessary. Pages that were once joined by staples and no longer are may be of interest in cases where it is alleged that pages have been removed or added or substituted from an original stapled bundle.

Paperclips often leave behind a telltale impression in the pages held together by them. These marks may provide evidence of how pages have been joined or added to a bundle, depending on the circumstances. Similarly,

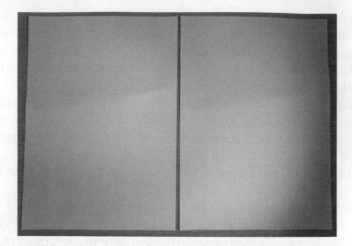

Figure 8.2 Two pieces of paper with similar crease patterns viewed under oblique light.

paper folds and creases may be present caused by, for example, the storage of the document (Figure 8.2). The creases need not be very marked and can be quite minor but nonetheless indicative that the pages have been together, and thus added pages may not show the creasing. Photocopy documents show the presence of staples and even staple holes and, depending on the circumstances, this may provide important evidence.

8.2.3 Punched holes and perforations

Punched holes may be part of the paper pad at the time of purchase or they can, of course, be added subsequently. The presence of such holes and their position and size may be measured and compared. In addition, photocopies of documents with punched holes often show the presence of the holes as a shadow on the photocopy document which, depending on the circumstances of the case, may be important (Figure 8.3).

Some official documents have perforations to facilitate manual splitting of part of the document. Counterfeiters will often attempt to reproduce the perforations by one means or another but are rarely able to reproduce them with the precision of the official document, as can be demonstrated by careful visual examination and, if necessary, measurement of the size and placement of the perforations.

8.3 The examination of written or machine-generated details

The handwriting, typescript or other printed details on a document can be altered or added to. The evidence for such alterations will often be similar to

Figure 8.3 Shadow staple holes (x3 approx.).

that required for a comparison between them, as described in Chapters 2–5. Essentially, the document examiner needs to be alert to the possibility that some details have been added or changed depending on the circumstances of the case. It is therefore impossible to generalise about what to look for in any particular case, but the key point is the need to be alert to the possibility that such an alteration might have been made and this in turn may be suggested by the circumstances of the case. For example, a set of accounts may have had amounts amended or a will may have had a paragraph or more added and so on. Changes may well be accompanied by changes in the materials used (see Sections 8.1 and 8.2) but that need not always be the case and so a careful examination of the handwriting or typeface, for instance, may still be required to show the alteration.

8.3.1 Erasures and obliterations

The erasure of ink from a document is rarely achieved without some disturbance to the paper surface. Erasure can be achieved by either physical abrasion using an eraser or by chemical treatment to effectively dissolve the ink. Physical abrasion will remove not only the ink but also some paper fibres, although the extent of disruption to the paper surface will depend on the care taken. Microscopic examination with side lighting will usually reveal the disturbed paper fibres and transmitted light may also show paper thinning in the area (Figure 8.4).

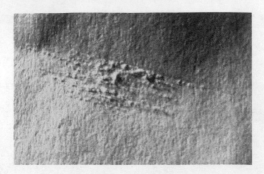

Figure 8.4   Oblique light view of an abraded document close up (x3 approx.).

The use of chemicals to remove ink from a document will often leave residual evidence of the chemical or traces of the ink. However, there is a need to protect some important documents (such as cheques) from chemical alteration and for this reason the paper used often has components in it that react with commonly used solvents that are used when attempting to remove ink in this way to produce a noticeable stain in the paper rendering the attempted alteration a failure. Some erasures may occur unintentionally, such as a document that is inadvertently 'washed' in a washing machine.

The document examiner's task is often two-fold in erasure cases. First, it is to show that an erasure has occurred and second, there may be evidence to reveal what the original entry was despite the attempted erasure. The evidence for erasure has been noted above, but deciphering of the original entry can be done by careful microscopy searching for any remnants of ink and, second, using the optical properties of the ink as described in Section 8.1.2 to enhance any traces of the ink still present.

An obliteration usually involves heavy over-inking of an entry with a second ink so as to render the first ink unreadable. Occasionally, the same ink is used for both the original entry and the crossing out and in this circumstance it may be very difficult to decipher the original entry. If the two inks used differ, then careful microscopy may reveal the original entry and the use of optical techniques may again assist by, for example, rendering the crossing out ink transparent to light at a particular wavelength (Figure 8.5).

If the obliteration is done using a correction fluid and then another entry written on top of the correction fluid, it is often possible to determine the original entry using transmitted light or careful microscopy. It is often worth examining the back of the sheet of paper as the original entry will be 'next to' the back of the sheet when viewed from behind and therefore not covered by the correction fluid (Figure 8.6).

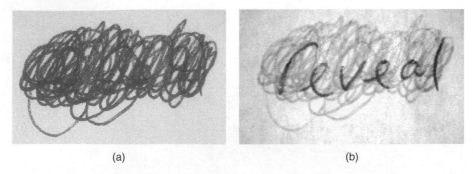

(a)   (b)

Figure 8.5   a and b. An obliterated entry before and after use of appropriate filters to reveal the original entry.

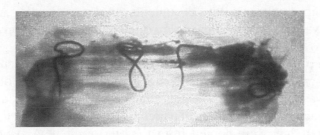

Figure 8.6   An entry covered with correction fluid viewed from behind the document illuminated with transmitted light. *(See insert for colour representation of the figure.)*

8.4   Copy documents

The examination of copy documents for evidence of alteration is inevitably more limited than the examination of original documents since information relating to paper and ink colour and the finer detail of handwriting or print comparison may be precluded. However, some cases require a comparison between different copy documents with a view to determining their relationship to one another. For example, one party might say that their copy document was derived from another party's copy or from an original document.

Such cases are often very difficult to examine (see also Chapter 4 for a discussion of the complex issues relating to copy documents). However, it is helpful if it is clear what is being alleged since it is often possible to show what has *not* happened rather than what has happened – 'This copy could not have come from that because ... ' as opposed to 'This copy might have come from that one or that one or ... '.

It is often possible to find evidence from other aspects of a document's production, such as the presence of staple holes or other marks that show

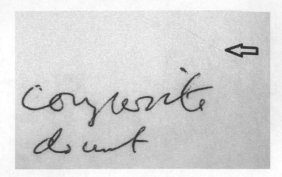

Figure 8.7   Showing a close up of a shadow line suggesting a composite document.

a relationship between copy documents and/or originals. As noted in Section 8.2, various marks on paper are often reproduced on copy documents and may be overlooked by the perpetrator as irrelevant.

One form of alteration case involving copies that used to occur frequently was the so-called cut-and-paste composite, in which part of a genuine document was combined with a non-genuine part of another document by physically placing the two pieces of paper together and copying them to make it appear that they were copied from the one original. A typical example might be that a genuine letterhead and signature would have different text added into the central part of a letter and copied. In such a case, the signature and letterhead are genuine but clearly the composite document is fraudulent. Evidence for such a composite often came from the shadow caused where the two pieces of paper overlapped, or other evidence such as a change of typeface if some details (such as a date at the top of the letter) were not covered over (Figure 8.7). The advent of the computer and scanner has made this task somewhat simpler.

8.5   Altering security documents

The complex materials and methods used to produce security documents have as one of their primary functions a requirement that making alterations is very difficult (the other function being that they are difficult to completely counterfeit). Attempts to alter a security document often revolve around the personalising details of that document, such as the page in a passport that identifies the holder. The success of the attempt, as indeed with any document alteration or counterfeit, depends on who it has to get past unnoticed. A passport used as a form of identity in a bank to open an account may be scrutinised by staff who do not have such in depth knowledge as, say, border officials at an airport, who in turn will not have the extensive training required of specialist security document examiners. Once a security document is examined by this latter group of experts, then there is every likelihood that evidence will be found to show whether it is genuine or whether it has been tampered with.

8.6 Case notes in alterations cases

Alterations cases often revolve around a comparison between the physical components of a document (see Chapter 6), sometimes requiring the use of specialist equipment (see Chapter 7), and so the note taking sections at the ends of these chapters is of relevance here.

Additionally, the context of a particular case and the specific allegations made, or the various alternatives that might reasonably apply in that case, will be unique. Hence, it is often a good idea to photocopy the relevant documents and highlight and annotate them showing what has been examined and what methods have been tried, for example. The crucial stage of the document examiner's role is to interpret the findings in a case, so while case notes must show all of the methods and equipment used and the results obtained, there must also be an explicit consideration of how this stacks up against competing possible explanations for the evidence. For example, it is important to avoid implying intent to a finding such as the use of a different ink to write part of a document – there might be a simple and innocent explanation with no intent to deceive.

The case notes should provide coherent links between the documents in question, the question being asked (such as what was the entry before it was obliterated), the methods used to answer the question, the evidence found and the interpretation of that evidence. That way, the expert will be able to recreate the examination at some point in the future if they need to give an explanation at an oral hearing.

8.7 Reports in alterations cases

Writing reports in alterations cases can often be very tricky and require some care over how the information is conveyed, especially if scientific equipment has been used. Where an alteration can be clearly photographed to show the evidence without distorting or misrepresenting it, it is worth considering adding a photograph to the report. It is generally unwise to make the report too technical as this will make it hard to understand by the non-specialist reader. If technical terms are unavoidable, then it may assist to have a glossary appended to the report or else to give a brief explanation of the term in brackets immediately after its use in the report.

Some alterations cases are very involved and may consist of many separate findings, such as a ledger sheet where entries have been changed, erased or obliterated. Rather than describe each one separately, it may be easier to tabulate the findings with perhaps two columns, one showing what is currently visible and the second column showing what was originally written. It is often difficult to decipher every single detail in an alteration case (similar to the problems with interpreting indented impressions – see Chapter 9). Where decipherments are uncertain, the character can be placed in brackets, or where it is indecipherable a hyphen can be used. Hence the entry 07(8)(2 or 3)- -4(1)77 might refer to a telephone number where some parts are uncertain. Document examiners should not over-interpret the evidence since an incorrect decipherment could thoroughly mislead an investigation.

The very variable nature of alterations cases makes it difficult to generalise any further as to how best they should be reported except to say that a clear and well structured layout (such as numbered paragraphs) will assist greatly in navigating the reader through the important aspects of the expert's findings.

Alterations examination: a worked example

In this section an example of how to approach a case and make notes is demonstrated. The worked example is intended to show a general process in terms of thinking and doing rather than the expectation that the reader will 'test' themselves to see if they can get the 'right' answer (although getting the 'right' answer could be regarded as a welcome bonus!).

It should be stressed that there are a number of different ways to make notes and the intention here is to show the kinds of issues that need to be considered and how these interrelate with the observation process leading to a conclusion.

Case circumstances

An agreement was allegedly signed on 11 January 2014 by various parties but a dispute arose and different versions of the agreement have been produced. Item 1 is one version that shows a date of 14 July 2014 which is significant in the context of this case. The date on item 1 was written by Henry Smith and he says that the date has not been altered and that the date as it appears now is how he wrote it at the time.

Purpose

To determine whether or not the date on item 1 has been altered.

Items submitted

Item 1: Agreement with date 14.7.14 (Figure 8.8).

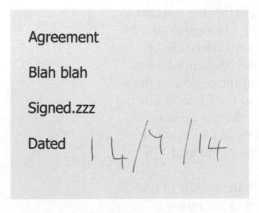

Figure 8.8 Worked example: Agreement, item 1.

Case notes

Observations	Thoughts
Microscopy shows an oily ink deposit with slight indentation into the paper surface typical of that associated with a ballpoint pen. Visual and microscopic examination shows no discernible difference in the ink colours.	What kind of pen has been used and is the ink similar?
After an exhaustive examination using various light sources and filters, no evidence that more than one ink is present was found.	Do instrumental techniques show any differences in the inks within the date?

If the date has been altered then either the same pen or another pen containing a similar ink was used. While this is often difficult to achieve, it can happen by chance and if the person that makes an alteration has access to the writing implements used then this makes such a situation more plausible. Note that even if an alteration is detected, there is no likelihood of saying when it was done.

Observations	Thoughts
Although the date contains a small amount of handwriting, there are two somewhat surprising features.	
• In the final '14' the horizontal part of the four is raised about half way up the adjacent numeral 1. In the '14' at the beginning the down stroke of the 4 is a similar length to the adjacent numeral 1 and the horizontal part is much lower than that of the final 4 in the date.	
• The 7 is not in the middle of the two slash strokes but rather is much nearer the first slash line. If the top of the 7 were not there, then the resulting numeral 1 would be roughly at the mid-point between the two slash lines. Further microscopy shows a possible break in the line between the top stroke and the down stroke, although this evidence is not absolutely conclusive as the pen may not have been inking properly.	
Examination of the reverse of the document does not show any difference in the pressure or embossing of the ink line so no further evidence from that line of thought.	If an alteration has been made it might have been made while the paper was resting on a different surface, so it is worth examining the reverse of the document.

At this point there is a suspicion that the date may have been altered, but to add weight to the evidence it might be helpful to examine some handwriting samples from Mr Smith containing numerals. As a result item 2 (Figure 8.9), a sample of dates written by him, is submitted for comparison. Thus a case that starts as purely one of establishing whether or not a document has been altered can require other evidence, in this case handwriting specimens, to help interpret what is found.

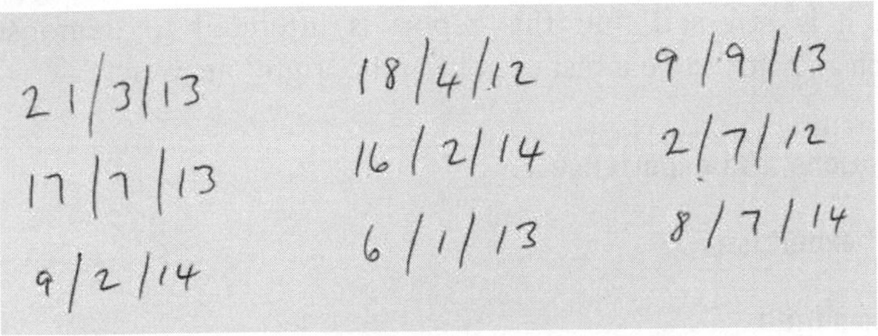

Figure 8.9 Worked example: Handwriting specimen.

Observations	Thoughts
The number 4 appears on three occasions and on each the horizontal part is above the lowest point of the adjacent number 1.	These specimens of handwriting show that indeed the date in question on item 1 is unusual in its appearance and they provide additional evidence to support the view that the questioned date has been altered.
The numeral 7 appears on four occasions and in none of them does it have the curved top found in item 1 and when present between the two slash lines it is approximately in the middle.	
	Alternative explanations:
	• The date has been altered possibly from 1/11/14.
	• The date has not been altered and the observed discrepancies are coincidental or accidental handwriting features.
	• On balance, the initial suspicions are confirmed by the handwriting specimens but the evidence is by no means strong with such a small amount of handwriting.

Report of Forensic Expert

(Again, it is stressed that this report is intended to demonstrate an approach and not to be a test of getting the 'right' answer.)

Qualifications and experience ...

Scope of expertise ...

Items examined

I have examined the following items at the instruction of (the investigating authority). They were received at the laboratory on (dates).

Item 1: Agreement

Item 2: Specimen of handwriting of Mr Smith

Purpose

I have examined the date on item 1 with a view to determining whether or not it has been altered and I have used the specimen handwriting of Mr Smith in item 2 to assist with this.

Findings

The date in question has been written with a similar ink throughout.

The first number 4 differs in its appearance from the second number 4. In particular, the horizontal part of the first 4 is lower than that of the second 4 suggesting the possibility that the first 4 has been altered from a number 1.

The number 7 is nearer the left slash line than the right slash line. If the top stroke of the 7 were not present the resulting number 1 would be roughly midway between the two slash lines.

The specimen handwriting of Mr Smith shows examples of the number 4 that are similar to the second number 4 in the date in question, but differ from the first number 4 in the questioned date. The format of the dates in the specimens shows that the number between the slash lines is written roughly midway between them.

Given the small amount of handwriting in the date in question, a definite opinion is not justified, but the observations noted do provide some limited evidence to show that, on balance, it is more likely than not the date on item 1 was altered probably from 11/1/14.

Summary

There is some limited evidence that the date on item 1 has been altered from 11/1/14.

References

Allen, M. J., & Rimmer, P. A. (1988). The dating of a will. *Journal of the Forensic Science Society*, 28(3), 199–203. doi: 10.1016/S0015-7368(88)72830-3.

Berger, C. E. H. (2009). Objective paper structure comparison through processing of transmitted light images. *Forensic Science International,* 192(1–3), 1–6. doi: 10.1016/j.forsciint.2009.07.004.

Biermann, C. J. (1996). *Handbook of Pulping and Papermaking*. London: Academic Press.

Causin, V., Casamassima, R., Marruncheddu, G., et al. (2012). The discrimination potential of diffuse-reflectance ultraviolet-visible-near infrared spectrophotometry for the forensic analysis of paper. *Forensic Science International*, 216(1–3), 163–167. doi:10.1016/j.forsciint.2011.09.015.

Green, J. A. (2012). Reliability of paper brightness in authenticating documents. *Journal of Forensic Sciences*, 57(4), 1003–1007. doi:10.1111/j.1556-4029.2012.02092.x.

Totty, R. N., Rimmer, P. A., & Steadman, R. K. (1987). Establishing the date of manufacture of a sheet of photocopy paper – a case example. *Journal of the Forensic Science Society*, 27(2), 81–88. doi: 10.1016/S0015-7368(87)72713-3.

9
Indented Impressions

One of the functions of forensic practice that is sometimes forgotten is that it can provide intelligence information *during* an investigation as opposed to providing evidence in the *aftermath* of a crime. One area in document examination where this is especially true is in the examination of documents for indented impressions of handwriting or signatures. A typical case situation might be where an anonymous document contains some kind of threat and the investigator wants to know the origin of the document. One avenue to explore is to see whether there are any indented impressions of handwriting on the document which were created when some other (upper) document was written whilst resting on the threatening (lower) document. If the handwriting on the upper document contains information such as a name or address or some other detail which indicates its origin, then that can provide useful intelligence information for the investigator to pursue as a possible line of enquiry.

When writing on a sheet of paper that is resting on at least one other sheet of paper (for example pages in a pad, but the pages need not be bound together) the act of writing *tends* to produce a groove in the paper caused by the pressure from the 'nib' (be it the ball in a ballpoint pen, the fibrous tip of a felt tip pen or the traditional nib of a fountain pen). The amount of pressure applied on the writing implement varies from one writer to another. The pressure is relayed to the paper surface via the nib of the writing implement. An inflexible hard nib, typified by the hard metal ball in a ballpoint pen, will relay the pressure to the paper surface and this translates to a noticeable groove in the paper corresponding to the line of writing. A flexible fibrous nib in a felt tip pen will tend to absorb the writing pressure and so produce little by way of a groove in the paper surface.

The act of writing with, for example, a ballpoint pen, will often cause an indentation in the sheet of paper below, indeed it may be detectable several sheets below. If the writing pressure is large then the indentation on the lower

Foundations of Forensic Document Analysis: Theory and Practice, First Edition. Michael Allen.
© 2016 John Wiley & Sons, Ltd. Published 2016 by John Wiley & Sons, Ltd.
Companion Website: www.wiley.com/go/allen/forensicanalysis

page may be visible to the naked eye. However, it is often the case that there is no visible indentation on the lower page and yet there is disruption to the surface, the nature of which enables the handwritten details to be visualised.

9.1 Visualising indented impressions

There are two main methods used to visualise indented impressions of handwriting. A third method, sometimes portrayed in fictional accounts, is to lightly apply a pencil to the paper surface to help show up any deep impressions – this is not an appropriate method and should not be used.

It should always be remembered that a piece of paper has two sides. In those instances in which there is only handwriting or other details on one side, that does not preclude the possibility that there are impressions of handwriting on the other side of the paper.

9.1.1 Electrostatic method

There are pieces of equipment on the market that enable the document examiner to examine the electrostatic properties of a sheet of paper (see also Box 9.1). The use of these electrostatic devices has been universal in the document laboratory since the late 1970s and they are regarded as an essential piece of equipment for the forensic document examiner.

The reason for making such examinations is that the act of writing on an upper page causes disruption to the surface of the lower page and, as noted above, this disruption can sometimes be so large as to cause a visible indentation. This is also accompanied by a disruption to the electrostatic properties of the paper and it is these that are exploited by the components and processes involved in an electrostatic examination (Daéid et al., 2008).

Box 9.1 Electrostatics

When two surfaces come into contact with one another, depending on the properties of the surfaces, it is possible for an electrostatic charge to be created between them. This happens because the negatively charged electrons that are present in the materials can move from a first surface to a second surface causing the first surface to acquire a positive charge (due to the loss of negative charge) and the second surface to acquire a negative charge.

The key point as far as the examination of indented impressions on paper is concerned is that paper can indeed form an electrostatic charge due to the chemical groups present in the cellulose and other components that make up the paper fibres. The effectiveness of this charging process may depend on the micro-structure of the paper surface because some papers may have different additives present to make them whiter or smoother, for example.

As with all electric phenomena, the underlying physics of electrostatics is complex and is governed by various mathematical relationships (such as Coulomb's Law and Gauss's Law). Nonetheless, as far as the document examiner is concerned, the effectiveness of the electrostatic examination of paper is affected by these laws in so much as such examinations work best under particular circumstances, such as moderately high relative humidity and when the contact between the surfaces has a frictional component. The long persistence of the electrostatic charge is consistent with the finding that electrostatic examinations can be carried out successfully on pieces of paper decades after the indented impressions were first made.

Visualising the impressions is a matter of first placing the piece of paper on the device. It is typically held on a sintered metal bed (which allows a vacuum to be drawn through it) and a vacuum pump is switched on to ensure a good contact between the piece of paper and the device. The paper is then covered with a sheet of thin, transparent polymer film that is capable of taking the electrostatic charge produced by passing a high voltage corona wire a few millimetres above the surface of the polymer film. This gives it a charge and then the film is exposed to a (black) powder that is attracted preferentially to the charged areas of the plastic that coincide with the electrostatic disruption to the paper surface. The toner application can be either via a cloud spraying device or by combining toner with microscopic glass beads that carry the toner on their surface and which can be cascaded over the document manually.

Whichever method is used, the end product is a polymer film with black powder attached in areas that correspond to the writing impressions, and thus the handwritten details can be deciphered. The electrostatic image can be preserved (for evidential purposes) by placing a transparent adhesive plastic sheet over the polymer and toner and lifting the whole from the electrostatic device.

The fact that such devices work has been shown innumerable times. What is less certain is the underlying science that explains why electrostatic techniques work (see also Box 9.1). The physical deformation (the 'groove' whether visible or not) itself may not be the cause; rather the disruption to the paper surface caused by frictional forces between the upper and lower sheets appears to cause changes to the electrostatic properties of the polymer and paper combination and this, together with the toner materials used to develop the image, leads to a decipherable trace (Daéid et al., 2008). This apparent need for a frictional component is consistent with the poor results obtained from impacting devices, such as typewriters, where the impression is created not by a moving object (such as a pen) but by a striking object, such as the typeface, as it impacts the paper with no lateral movement.

Furthermore, good quality papers tend to yield the best results in terms of a decipherable trace, but if the paper is too heavily processed (such as a glossy magazine cover) the fibres on the surface may not be so readily disturbed leading to a poor result. Similarly, rough paper surfaces (such as blotting paper) tend not to give good results. The overall physical smoothness of the paper is also important such that, for example, heavily creased or crumpled paper will tend not to lie flat on the metal bed leading to poor contact between the paper and the polymer film.

High relative humidity (see also Box 9.2) is also often beneficial to electrostatic paper examinations (D'Andrea et al., 1996) (see also Box 9.2).

Box 9.2 Humidity

Humidity is often referred to in absolute terms or in relative terms. Humidity refers to the amount (mass) of water vapour in a given volume of gas (usually the atmosphere). The amount of water vapour changes as the temperature or the pressure of the atmosphere changes. At a given temperature and pressure, the atmosphere can hold only so much water vapour at which point it is described as being saturated. The amount of water at saturation goes up with increasing temperature and pressure.

Relative humidity relates to the humidity at a given temperature and is a measure of the amount of water vapour present in comparison to the amount of water vapour that would reach saturation at that temperature.

For most situations where humidity is a factor, it is the relative humidity that is more relevant since it is a measure at a fixed temperature. In the electrostatic examination of paper for indented impressions of handwriting, the environment in which the devices and the pages for examination are held can be controlled for temperature and relative humidity in an attempt to achieve optimal conditions for visualising the impressions (D'Andrea et al., 1996). In the absence of an environmentally controlled room, the documents for examination can be placed in a humid environment (such as a closed humidification chamber) and the temperature and humidity can be measured using a hygrometer.

The very close control of the environmental conditions is generally not critical to the success or failure of the electrostatic examination for impressions (except possibly with very faint impressions, which may not be detected at all if the conditions are not optimal). Rather, the closer to optimal circumstances that can be achieved, the greater the likelihood of improving the decipherability of the trace in terms of the contrast between the impressions and the background.

When examining a piece of paper on which there is visible ink-written hand-writing, such handwriting will often appear as white on the electrostatic trace. Also, when examining the 'reverse' of a piece of paper that has either original ink-written handwriting or impressions of handwriting on the 'front' these may well show up on the electrostatic trace but in mirror image orientation.

9.1.2 Secondary impressions

Not only can electrostatic devices be used for visualising impressions caused by the straightforward act of writing on an upper sheet of paper, they can also be used in a number of related situations. If a first sheet of paper has indented impressions of handwriting on it, and that sheet of paper comes into contact with a second piece of paper which does not initially have those impressions, then the very physical contact between the two sheets can sometimes lead to the 'impressions being transferred' to the second sheet, forming what are often referred to as secondary impressions (Barr et al., 1996).

9.1.3 Determining the sequence of handwriting and impressions

In some case situations a document can bear handwriting and also indented impressions of some other handwritten details, and a question may arise over whether the handwriting visible on the sheet or the impressions were present first. Sequencing handwriting and impressions of handwriting requires that they cross over at some points. An electrostatic examination shows that where the ink of some handwriting is already present on the surface of the paper and indented impressions are then created on that same sheet, the usual dark line of the handwriting impression on the electrostatic trace is interrupted by the presence of the ink (Radley, 1993) – see also Figure 9.1.

As noted in Chapter 3, signatures may be traced in such a way as to create a visible groove in the paper which is subsequently inked in to produce the forgery. If the inking in stage is done carefully, it may be difficult to detect the initial groove. An electrostatic trace of the area associated with the signature may show the presence of the groove and help to demonstrate how the forgery was created.

9.1.4 Examining multiple-page documents

Electrostatic examinations tend to work best if only one sheet is examined at a time on the device. This creates a problem if the document consists of multiple pages. If the pages are bound into a book then the page to be examined can be isolated and the remaining pages carefully moved away so that the page can be held on the device and covered with the polymer film. This therefore

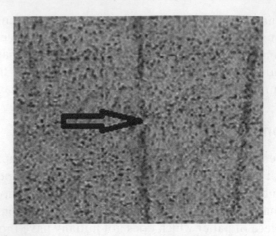

Figure 9.1 The dark grey line is typical of that produced by an impression and the pale tramlined line (running from bottom left to top right) is typical of that produced by an inkline on the paper. Where they cross (arrowed) any break in the lines may indicate whether the impressions were present on the page before the ink or vice versa (×3 approx.)

requires two people, one to hold the document in place and one to carry out the examination.

Alternatively pages can be cut from a document but only if permission to do so has been obtained from the investigator. If this approach is used, then it is important to identify the sequence of pages in the book before any are removed, for instance by writing a sequence of page numbers in the corner of each page.

Some pads are held together by spiral bindings. It is possible to manipulate these spirals by rotating them so that they can be removed. If this is done, again pages need to be numbered before dismantling the pad and permission from the investigator is needed.

9.1.5 Deciphering electrostatic traces

The interpretation of an electrostatic trace can be straightforward when there is good contrast between the dark toner (showing the indented handwriting) and the general background (see, for instance, Figure 9.3 in the Worked Example at the end of this chapter). However, in some cases the handwriting is shown very faintly and it may be difficult or impossible to decipher the details with certainty. When deciphering faint impressions, it is important to try to avoid cognitive bias such as: Do the impressions say such and such? If there is uncertainty over what the impressions say then alternatives should be reported. For example: The impressions can be deciphered to read '0878 (5 or 6) (1 or 7) 33'. Similarly, where there are impressions present but they cannot be deciphered then their presence should be reported but their content left undeciphered.

Deciphering of words, in particular, is often context dependent. For example the letters 'Chris' at the start of a longer word may be very clear but the ending of the word may not be clear for some reason. However, if the surrounding words are concerned with Christmas then there is an inevitable temptation to 'fill in the gaps' and to read the whole word as Christmas. In these cases, care must be taken not to over-interpret what is seen and a common-sense view taken as to whether the unclear element is at least consistent with any filling in (for example if the word in fact was Christopher and not Christmas that would probably be obvious). Such deciphering is similar to the process of reading handwriting that is poorly formed and semi-illegible but which can be made sense of by the capacity of the human brain to 'work out' what has been written, not from each letter but from our knowledge of words, spelling, context and use of language.

As noted above, impressions of handwriting will often be detectable on not just the page immediately below that being written on but also on the next pages, commonly the third or fourth pages and sometimes beyond even those. If each page in a pad is written on, this means that on, say, the fifth page in the pad, there may be fairly clear impressions of handwriting from the handwriting on the fourth page, somewhat fainter impressions from the handwriting on the third page, even fainter impressions from the handwriting on the second page and perhaps yet fainter impressions from the handwriting on the first page. An electrostatic examination of the fifth page may reveal several sets of impressions from the pages above and these may well overlap one another making them very hard to disentangle to decipher. It may also be difficult to decide which impressions go together. For example, if there is a name and a telephone number revealed by the trace, were they written on the same sheet of paper (therefore suggesting an association between the name and the number) or were they in fact written on different sheets (and therefore do not necessarily suggest an association between the name and the number) and coincidentally show up roughly in the same place on the trace? Again, the human brain's capacity for language can assist and may suggest which entries might go together and this, taken with any differences in intensity of the impressions revealed by the electrostatic trace, might help make sense of the pattern of evidence.

When impressions are overlapping and difficult to decipher, it is sometimes a good idea to give the electrostatic trace showing the impressions to the investigator to see whether there are any details that appear to be significant to them. Of course, this again risks cognitive bias as the investigator is effectively looking for impressions that fit in with his or her preconceived ideas of what might be there, so it is essential that the eventual deciphering of any details of interest is done by the document examiner who can put forward any alternative interpretations where there is uncertainty and avoid misrepresenting the evidence.

Occasionally the revealed impressions are very faint and cannot be deciphered readily. One possibility is to carry out a second electrostatic examination and to superimpose the two traces obtained with the view of getting a darker combined trace.

9.2 Oblique light

When examining a document for impressions of indented handwriting, the use of electrostatic devices is often the first process to be considered by the document examiner. However, there are some circumstances where the use of oblique light is more effective. The oblique light method for detecting impressions requires simply the illumination of the paper surface with a strong light source (such as light from a fibre optic) shone at a grazing angle to the paper surface (Figure 9.2). Any reasonably deep (visible) impression grooves in the paper will cast a shadow due to the grazing angle of the light, which can be photographed as a record of the evidence. The deciphering can be done at the time of the examination but the photographic record should show, as far as possible, those details that are deciphered.

As noted in Section 9.1, deep impressions that produce easily visible indentations in the paper surface are not always well visualised using electrostatic devices. By their very nature, indentations that can be seen with oblique light vary in depth from barely detectable to very obvious. The less deep impressions are very likely to also be visualised using an electrostatic device. This is important when the expert is confronted by a lot of pages to examine (such as a thick pad of paper) and when searching for any pages that might

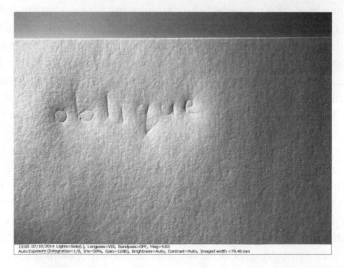

Figure 9.2 Indented impressions revealed using an oblique light source to produce shadows created by the deep impression.

have any impressions at all. By their very nature, writing pads can be written on at any page and pages can be readily removed, so to examine every single page using the electrostatic method would be very time consuming and sometimes time is critical in an investigation – such as in a kidnapping. Using an oblique light source to (relatively) quickly examine each page of a 200-page pad for any faint signs of impressions might enable attention to be focused on a small proportion of the pages for further electrostatic examination – broadly, an oblique light examination may take seconds per page, an electrostatic examination will take several minutes per page.

As already noted, oblique light is often the only method that enables deep impressions of indented handwriting to be visualised and recorded. Impressions caused by other factors, such as typescript, are again best examined using oblique light (see Section 9.1). One case situation that occurs now and again is the examination of very glossy paper, such as is found on magazine covers. Electrostatic techniques do not always work well with such paper and oblique light is made more difficult by the considerable reflection of the light from the shiny surface. If the impressions are deep enough, it may be possible to take a cast of the impressions using a very fine-grained casting material of the type widely used by forensic practitioners that examine toolmark impressions. When dry, the cast can be viewed with oblique light to emphasise the impressions, which are now in relief to the background, to assist with the deciphering process.

Recording impressions viewed with oblique light is done photographically. Getting the ideal lighting angle is important to make the impressions as clear as possible. If, for example, a whole page of A4 paper bears impressions, it may be difficult to cast a strong enough light at an ideal angle to record the impressions across the entire page in one photograph. Instead, it may be better to photograph several areas of the page, making sure that the photographs record slightly overlapping regions of the page so as not to omit any details. The recording of the impressions serves not only as a record of what the document examiner found but also allows such evidence to be presented to others at a later date in a court hearing, for instance.

9.3 Case notes in indented impressions cases

The primary purpose of notes in such cases is to record what has been done and what has been deciphered. All findings, including negative findings, should be recorded. For example, the use of oblique light may be tried and may well reveal nothing visible, but the process and outcome can be briefly noted. If an electrostatic method is used, then the humidity and temperature conditions can be recorded. It is essential that an electrostatic trace can be linked back to the relevant document from which it is derived by appropriate labelling of the trace.

The deciphering stage can be carried out in a number of ways. For example, a photocopy of the trace can be annotated and the deciphered details written adjacent to each entry. It is essential that any uncertainty in the deciphering is clearly recorded and that this corresponds to the way that the results are presented in any final report or statement. If it is unclear which deciphered details belong together, then it is essential that this is indicated in the manner in which they are represented in the written report to avoid misleading the investigator.

It is a common occurrence to carry out an electrostatic examination of a document and not observe any evidence of impressions of handwriting. Such negative findings can also be retained since it is a record of what was found and if called into question subsequently, the trace can be produced as evidence of what was *not* found.

In cases in which oblique light has produced evidence, a photograph of the impressions should be obtained as noted above. In some cases the oblique light findings and the electrostatic findings may complement one another with some details better revealed by one process and other details by the second process. Which details are best revealed by which process also needs to be recorded.

9.4 Reports in indented impressions cases

Reporting cases involving indented impressions of handwriting are generally straightforward since they require just a description of the details deciphered. The main issue is to make sure that any uncertainties about specific elements of the deciphering are clearly indicated (see also Section 9.1.5). If a piece of equipment is used to visualise the impressions then this needs to be mentioned in the report, but it is not normally necessary to describe how the machine works.

If the evidence is particularly difficult to decipher, it may be worth considering scanning any visualised impressions and including these images in the report to assist the reader in interpreting the findings.

Impressions examination: a worked example

In this section an example of how to approach a case and make notes is demonstrated. The worked example is intended to show a general process in terms of thinking and doing, rather than the expectation that the reader will 'test' themselves to see if they can get the 'right' answer (although getting the 'right' answer could be regarded as a welcome bonus!).

It should be stressed that there are a number of different ways to make notes, and the intention here is to show the kinds of issues that need to be considered and how these interrelate with the observation process leading to a conclusion.

Case circumstances

A hold up note was left behind at the scene.

Purpose

To examine the note with a view to finding and deciphering any impressions of handwriting present on the note.

Items submitted

Item 1: Hold up note

Case notes

Observations	Thoughts
An examination using electrostatic apparatus is carried out with the temperature and humidity noted. The cascade application was used. Figure 9.3 shows the resulting trace.	The note is written on a plain piece of paper. Some faint impressions are visible to the naked eye but these will be best visualised using an electrostatic technique.
The details visualised on the trace are clear and can be deciphered as follows: 24 Sherry 48 Lemo 12 To(---) wa(t)er 24 Whisky	Is the trace clear enough to decipher some or all of the details with confidence? The third entry is partly obscured by the handwriting on the hold up note. Although it probably reads 'Tonic water' it is safest to indicate the uncertain details using brackets.

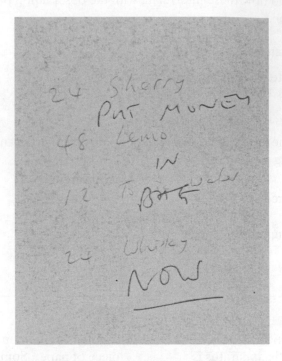

Figure 9.3   Worked example: Electrostatic trace from the hold up note.

Report of Forensic Expert

(Again, it is stressed that this report is intended to demonstrate an approach and not to be a test of getting the 'right' answer.)

Qualifications and experience ...

Scope of expertise ...

Items examined

I have examined the following items at the instruction of (the investigating authority). They were received at the laboratory on (dates).

Item 1: Note left at scene

Purpose

I have examined the note, item 1, with a view to deciphering any impressions of handwriting that may be present.

Findings

There are impressions of handwriting on item 1 which I have deciphered to read as follows. Entries in brackets are uncertain.

24 Sherry

48 Lemo

12 To(---) wa(t)er

24 Whisky

Summary

Item 1 bears impressions of handwriting as noted above.

References

Barr, K. J., Pearse, M. L., & Welch, J. R. (1996). Secondary impressions of writing and ESDA-detectable paper-paper friction. *Science & Justice*, 36(2), 97–100. doi:10.1016 /S1355-0306(96)72573-X.

D'Andrea, F., Mazzella, W. D., Khanmy, A., & Margot, P. (1996). The effects of the relative humidity and temperature on the efficiency of the ESDA process, *International Journal of Forensic Document Examiners*, 2(3), 209–213.

Daéid, N., Hayes, K., & Allen, M. (2008). Investigations into factors affecting the cascade developer used in ESDA – A review. *Forensic Science International*, 181(1–3), 1–9. doi:DOI: 10.1016/j.forsciint.2008.09.003.

Radley, R. W. (1993). Determination of sequence of writing impressions and ball pen inkstrokes using the esda technique. *Journal of the Forensic Science Society*, 33(2), 69–72. doi:10.1016/S0015-7368(93)72983-7.

10
Dating Documents

One of the most frequently asked questions, but one that is most difficult to answer, is: Can the date of production of a document be determined? The reason that this request is so common is that often documents are created at some time other than their purported date to justify some particular claim. For example, an agreement may be drafted but given a date that is years in the past to justify some financial gain or other.

It perhaps should be made clear at this point that dating a document does not refer to determining the actual day on which a document was produced! Absolute dating is often an approximate term, for example finding evidence that a document was produced after a particular date or period ('the questioned document was produced after 1950 because … '). Relative dating is where
a document's time of production can be established in relation to some other document's production ('the questioned page was written before/after some other page').

The possibility of dating when a document was produced will be significantly influenced by the nature of the document concerned. In this chapter, dating options will be considered for a number of document production methods, starting with a simple handwritten document.

10.1 Dating handwriting

The dating of handwriting (as opposed to the dating of ink on paper) is a possibility that depends upon the time factor in a particular case. Handwriting changes in a given writer are most rapid in the young (typically those under the age of about 20), the elderly (extremely variable, but typically by about 70 years of age handwriting may start to deteriorate), and in those with certain medical conditions that affect handwriting production (see Chapter 2).

Foundations of Forensic Document Analysis: Theory and Practice, First Edition. Michael Allen.
© 2016 John Wiley & Sons, Ltd. Published 2016 by John Wiley & Sons, Ltd.
Companion Website: www.wiley.com/go/allen/forensicanalysis

The likelihood of being able to date handwriting production will be considerably affected by the time gap involved. For example, say the time gap in question was five years with a document having been written five years before (or after) it purportedly was written. If a document was alleged to have been written when the writer was aged either 13 or 18 then it may well be possible to reach a conclusion providing suitable samples are available. Such a five-year gap when comparing handwriting from a person aged 40 and when they were aged 35, however, is much less likely to yield any notable differences as handwriting at these ages is generally stable and unlikely to have demonstrably changed. Then again, a five-year gap between 75 and 80 years of age in a writer may well reveal a notable deterioration, particularly if associated with medical conditions such as the onset of Parkinson's disease.

If instead of five years the gap is one year or six months or one month, then clearly as the gap decreases the less likely it will be that there is any evidence of change, even in younger and older people whose handwriting may alter more rapidly. Conversely, if the time gap at issue were to increase from 5 years to 10, 20 or more years, then the chances of finding differences will increase across all age groups.

The most important factor in such cases is obtaining reliable handwriting samples, as the date on which they were written is crucial to being able to carry out the relevant examination. Finding specimen documents written in the past, especially several years previously, and which bear dates or whose date of production can be approximated (for example in school books or diaries) is by no means readily achieved in many cases. Also, when dealing with medical conditions, the nature of the illness and the taking of any medication (which may lead to short-term improvements in handwriting movement control) are relevant factors to consider, and it may be that expert medical input is needed to confirm the impact that the condition has on a person's ability to write.

As described in Chapter 2, the way in which a person writes is influenced by their educational experiences, which in turn vary in time and place with different styles being taught in different countries and with more styles replacing older ones. This creates the possibility that allegedly historical documents may be written in a style that was not used at that time.

10.2   Dating ink

Dating when an ink-written document was created has been extensively studied. For a review of much of the research, Brunelle's book listed in Further Reading in the Preface gives a lot more detail than can be given here.

Perhaps the simplest approach is to determine the nature of the components present in an ink in order to determine whether those components were available at the relevant time. For instance, if a document is dated 1928 but was written with a ballpoint pen, then that would not be possible since the ballpoint pen was not invented and available until a few years later. Likewise, as the components of ink have become more complex over time, if it is known when a certain component was first used then this gives an earliest date of availability for inks incorporating it. The difficulty with such an approach is that much of the information relating to the introduction of different ink components is commercially sensitive and is not easily discovered (Weyermann et al., 2012). It is possible instead to collect samples of inks and analyse them and thereby create a database of inks and link this to information on when they were first available. This resource can then be used to compare questioned inks against the database in an attempt to determine its (approximate) date of production or to at least determine when it could not have been produced. Indeed, for a time various tags (such as rare earth elements not normally found in inks) were added to inks at different times to make dating them more feasible, but this had modest uptake with the manufacturers.

There are in principle two types of ink dating question that can be asked: (i) When was the ink placed on the document? (ii) When was the ink of this entry placed on the document *in relation to* other entries (usually on the same document)? In other words, absolute dating and relative dating of ink, respectively. There are two important types of confounding factor in ink dating problems that centre on:

(i) The ink and paper used at the time. Inks are complex mixtures made from different components and these may also be affected by the nature of the paper (made from different materials and having different physical properties such as absorbency) onto which the ink is placed.

(ii) The way in which the documents are stored after they have been created. At one extreme, an ink-written document left on a sunny window sill will be affected very differently to a document that is filed away soon after creation in amongst many other documents in a closed filing cabinet.

Despite the difficulties, much research has been carried out addressing the ink dating problem, particularly the relative dating since, in most cases, any confounding factors should apply equally to all parts of a document (assuming it was created with the same materials and stored in similar conditions).

The drying of ink on the page is perhaps an obvious theoretical starting point for the dating of ink. Some components of ink evaporate relatively quickly or else diffuse into the paper, whereas other components will be absorbed and adsorbed by the paper substrate (Weyermann et al., 2012) (see also Box 10.1). As a consequence of the various types of process involved, the drying of ink on paper is a complex process (Cantu, 2012).

Gel pen inks (which are water-based but which contain a mix of other components such as glycerol, ethylene glycol and diethylene glycol) were studied by Li and colleagues using gas chromatography (Li et al., 2014) showing that some volatile components of the inks evaporate rapidly over the first days and that artificial ageing causes loss of the volatile components in a matter of hours.

Box 10.1 Evaporation, diffusion, absorption and adsorption

The components of ink serve a number of functions that are designed to ensure that ink flows from a pen onto the paper and that once on the paper the ink dries at a suitably rapid rate and remains stable on the page under normal environmental storage conditions.

The physical properties of the ink's components together with the nature of the paper onto which it is written will determine their subsequent behaviour. The most volatile components will evaporate fairly rapidly and hence will be lost to the environment (usually to the atmosphere).

Some components of the ink will remain in the paper but will migrate away from the original site of the ink line by a process of diffusion in which molecules physically move through the solid medium of the paper structure. Some components of the ink are absorbed into the structure of the paper. In these two instances, the ink components do not become attached to or part of the paper but remain separate from the paper, albeit closely associated with its structure.

Some components of ink will, over time, become adsorbed by the paper fibres, a process that effectively means that these components become attached to and part of the paper itself.

The movement of ink components will vary according to many factors, including the particular components actually present in a particular ink, the amount of ink deposited (the thickness of the layer of ink which is a reflection of the amount of pressure applied to the pen by the writer), the width of the ink line (determined by the size of the nib or ball in a ballpoint pen), and the shape of the written character (for example a straight line – where ink will tend to move away from it evenly, compared to a small enclosed loop where ink components may move away outward from the loop but also move inwardly towards the centre of the loop and accumulate there) (Weyermann et al., 2012).

Ink dating methods have focused on all of these processes since in principle they offer different approaches to establishing how long the ink has been on the paper.

The drying process not only leads to the loss of the more volatile components of the ink, it is also associated with changes in the physical properties of other components, particularly the resins present, which may tend to harden and thus become more difficult to extract from the document. This leads to the idea that the longer the ink has been on the document, the more difficult it is to extract using a solvent. An extension of this idea is that at some point the changes to the ink will reach an end point and stop. Hence, if this end point could be determined for the ink on a particular document, the extent of the ink's time passage towards that end point would be an indication of how long the ink had been on the document. From this comes the idea of what amounts to the artificial ageing of the document. By warming the document under controlled conditions the natural process of ink drying can be sped up to reach its end point. If the extractability of the ink 'now' (*before* the document is artificially aged) is determined (perhaps giving a value of X) and this is compared to the extractability *after* artificial ageing (giving a value Y), then X should be greater than Y and by an amount that indicates how far short the ink is of reaching its end point.

Using the artificial ageing approach requires some knowledge of the *rate of change* of extractability of ink from a document. Many studies have found that the process is not linear but rather appears to be exponential. In other words, the rate of change in extractability is rapid to begin with (essentially meaning that many of the changes due to drying are relatively rapid over days and weeks) and that thereafter the changes in extractability are much slower over subsequent months and years, with the proviso that, for a given ink and document, the rates of change will depend on the confounding factors noted above (Weyermann et al., 2012).

The many methods of ink comparison have often been employed to address the ink dating issue as well as the more common problem of distinguishing between different inks (see Chapter 7 and Box 10.2). The important point is that, as for any technique, the methods used should be thoroughly tested and validated before being used in the forensic arena and that uncertainties caused by the potential confounding factors of materials used and storage conditions must be factored in as potential sources of error. Just as with other document dating problems, the time gaps that are relevant to a particular case will have a major impact on the usefulness (and especially the reliability) of evidence from ink dating methods.

Box 10.2 Ink dating methods

The many methods that can be used to compare inks can also be used to address the ink dating problem. Some of the methods used in ink dating are given here and a description of the methods can be found in Chapter 7. One important and common theme in the published literature is a need to exercise considerable caution when interpreting results in ink ageing problems because of the many confounding factors involved.

The following is a sample of papers from the literature. That by Ezcurra and colleagues (2010) is a useful starting point that surveys not only recent developments but also has a broader historical perspective as well.

- Ezcurra et al. (2010) is a review paper that surveys many of the published methods used in ink dating both in terms of the analytical techniques used and the methodologies by which they are applied.

- Gas chromatography and UV-visible spectroscopy. Gel and rollerball inks were analysed both for their relative and absolute ageing by Xu et al. (2006).

- Aginsky (1993) found that some components of ink will become less readily extracted the longer that they have been on the paper.

10.3   Dating paper (and other related materials)

Paper is a complex material with many different organic and inorganic components (see Chapter 6). The (approximate) date of the introduction of some components into paper manufacturing may be known and can provide information on the earliest date on which such papers could have been available. A well-known example was in the case of the forged Hitler diaries in the 1980s. Optical brighteners were first introduced into the paper industry in the late 1940s, and yet the diaries, allegedly describing events before his death in 1945, were in part written on paper containing such brighteners. Indeed, not only the paper but also other components of the binding of the diaries were shown to have not been available until years later.

Paper manufacturers generally keep records of what materials they use to make their papers and other information relating to production, such as the dates on which watermarks are introduced. Such background information can be a way of determining when a piece of paper was made. The dates on which different watermarks were introduced by a paper manufacturer have enabled the date of production of a will to be determined (Allen & Rimmer, 1988). Similarly, the use of a particular set of pulp fibres in a paper's manufacture again led to the dating of its production by cross-checking with the records at the paper mill (Totty et al., 1987).

Despite the occasional success in dating paper and related products, such successes are rare because most materials used in document production are widely available and remain unchanged over long periods of time. New products, however, do provide potential for dating documents and, together with manufacturer's records, there may be a chance of a successful forensic investigation. That said, the vast majority of paper is featureless (for example having no watermark) so identifying the manufacturer in the first place is extremely difficult.

10.4   Dating typescript and other mechanical processes

The fonts used in typewriters changed over time as new typefaces were introduced. The rate of newly conceived styles increased rapidly once computers became more commonplace. But the fact that typestyles have a date when they first were available again provides a possible mechanism for dating documents.

As with other dating methods, the longer the gap between the purported date of production and the actual date of production (assuming that indeed the document is fraudulent), the better the chance that there will be something wrong about the fake document. The date on which a particular typeface became available is likely to be difficult to establish with any precision and indeed its availability may vary from place to place since many products may be launched in one country before becoming available elsewhere, for example.

At a more general level, different technologies have been introduced over time, although again they will not have a precise launch date but rather became more and more widely available. For example, inkjet technology was introduced during the late 1970s, so a document dated 1965 that was inkjet printed is unlikely to be genuine. Further, inkjet technology has improved over time with, for example, ever smaller droplet sizes becoming available, so if the drop size can be calculated (with reference to the dot size on the paper) it may be possible to show that a document bearing a date of, say, 1985 could not have been produced at that time because the dot sizes are too small; in other words, the quality of the technology used to produce the suspect document was not available at the time when it was purportedly created.

Printing devices will tend to become damaged with use (see Chapter 4). Any change over time provides the potential for being able to demonstrate a chronological sequence of changes in documents produced on a device over time. For example, a brand new typewriter or computer printer will probably produce well-aligned, clear typed output, but over time with much use characters may misalign or become damaged or various components may malfunction such that the typed product is no longer 'perfect'. Documents produced during this period of deterioration are a record of the changes and if they are dated (or their date of production is known) then this becomes a reference chronology against which a suspect document can be compared. A case example that shows this made use of the fact that the gradual break up of a single letter (lower case k) on a printwheel typing element occurred over a period of months and the chronology that could be established enabled the suspect document's date of production to be established (or more precisely a period of time during which it must have been produced) and this did not correspond to the date on the suspect document (Hardcastle, 1986).

As noted in Chapter 4, some changes that occur in mechanical devices such as printers and copiers may be transient. For example, servicing may improve a defective copier or replacing a printer cartridge may change the appearance of a computer printer's output. However, as defect marks on a photocopier, for example, accumulate over time, they will create a chronology that can in principle be used to date when a questioned document was produced on that copier during this period of time. Such factors must be taken into account when assessing the evidence in relation to establishing reliable chronological sequences of documents.

10.5   Dating pages from a pad or stack of paper

The examination of pages in such multi-page documents is not perhaps strictly speaking a dating issue as it is normally considered, but rather it is concerned with showing when pages were created in relation to one another.

10.5.1   Impressions of handwriting

A suspect document can either bear impressions of handwriting that come from some other document (A) or the handwriting from a suspect document can appear as impressions on some other document (B). Which of these two situations occurs will be dependent upon the presence of sheets of paper in a stack or pad at the time. If either of the other documents (A or B or both) bears a true date (in other words the written date is the actual date that the document was written), then it might be possible to show whether the suspect document was written before or after one or other of A or B by following the approach described for sequencing handwriting and impressions of handwriting in Section 9.1.3 of Chapter 9 to determine whether the handwriting or the impressions of handwriting were created first on the page.

This complicated situation can be illustrated with a short example. An invoice is written out to cover up a financial fraud. The invoice is from a pad of invoices and the suspect invoice dated 1 March is number 20 in the pad. Examination of invoice number 21 is dated 1 July in the same year (its true date of being written) and it shows impressions of handwriting from the writing on invoice number 20 and these impressions overlap in some places with the actual handwriting on the invoice number 21. An electrostatic examination of invoice number 21 indicates that the handwriting on it was written *before* the impressions were created (from the handwriting invoice number 20). This would then show that invoice number 20 was written at some time after invoice number 21 was written out, in other words at some point after 1 July and not on 1 March.

10.5.2 Ink transfer

If an upper document is written on a pad resting directly on a sheet below that already bears handwriting, then the pressure applied during the production of the handwriting on the upper document may cause some of the ink on the page beneath to be transferred onto the reverse of the upper document. The areas of ink transfer will correspond to points when the writing on the upper sheet crossed the handwriting on the lower sheet. If such ink transfer occurs and can be demonstrated, it shows that the upper document was written at some time after the lower document was written out.

10.5.3 Multipage documents

Some documents consist of many pages and are written on pages that form a stack or (if bound) a pad of paper. In such cases, a series of pages are supposedly written in sequence such that page one was written out whilst resting on page two and then put to one side when the page was full, then page two was written on whilst resting on page three and so on down the stack. An example might be simply writing a long letter over several pages on lined paper from a typical A4 pad. Another example would be taking down a written record of some kind on pages in a stack, and over the years the prime example of this has been police notes of interview. If at some point the handwritten record is changed for some reason and a sheet of paper discarded and re-written, then this will be apparent from an examination of the impressions of handwriting on the relevant sheets. For example, if a mistake is made half way down page four and this page is discarded and a new page four is written on the next available sheet in the stack, then examination for impressions of handwriting on this new page four may show the content of the discarded page four.

10.6 Sequencing

The order in which the many different media that can be used to produce a document were placed on the document may be important to establish (for simplicity, all media will be referred to as using inks in this section). Given the many ways of creating a document (ranging from use of pens to typewriters and printers and printing to stampmarks) it is not surprising that the methods to determine their sequence of placement on a document vary across those described in Chapter 7, although some techniques have been developed to specifically address the sequencing problem in some cases.

The interaction between the first and second ink will depend on two key factors. First is the nature of the inks, whether they are water based or oil based (Ozbek et al., 2014) or some other medium (such as toner). Second, the time gap between when the first ink is placed on the document and the second ink is then used will affect the extent to which the first ink has had an opportunity to dry. In terms of the forensic examination, a third parameter is the time lapse between writing with the inks and the examination being made. There are, therefore, many potential problems when examining such cases and great caution is needed when interpreting the observations.

10.6.1 Ballpoint ink and ballpoint ink

Perhaps the most frequently encountered sequence problem is where two ballpoint pen ink lines cross (for example, where a body of text intersects an associated signature and the signatory alleges that some of the text has been added after the document was signed). A microscopic examination of the points where the ink lines intersect will rarely give a clear indication as to which line is first, and particular care needs to be taken when the two ink lines are of different intensity – as the darker ink will appear to be written over the lighter ink but this may be an optical illusion – so this observation should be treated with extreme caution.

A method that has been developed specifically for this type of problem involves the use of a high gloss card that is placed over the intersecting ink lines and heavy pressure applied, which has the effect of lifting some of the ink from the page onto the card (Mathyer & Pfister, 1984).

10.6.2 Stamp pad inks and other media

The interaction between the liquid ink from a stamp pad and other media, such as pen inks and toner, will depend to some extent on the amount of mixing between the first and second inks. Raman spectroscopy and high performance thin layer chromatography have been used with some success to determine the sequences in some instances (Raza & Saha, 2013).

10.6.3 Toner and other inks

The molten powder-like nature of toner from a photocopier or laser printer has the effect of the toner sitting on the surface of the paper with very little of the material absorbed into the paper surface. One method to examine the intersection is by using microscopy to look at the sheen and reflection of the toner, for example, and the effect of the ink on these properties (Saini et al., 2009). Caution may be needed in some instances, however, as when a liquid ink, such as from a gel pen, is applied before or after toner, the ink tends to seep through, giving the appearance that the toner was applied after the ink (Montani et al., 2012). Rather than looking at the inks themselves, it is possible to examine the micro-topography of the paper surface where the groove of the ink line and the toner material intersect using laser profilometry (a method of looking at the microscopic 'hills and valleys' present in a small area of the paper surface) (Montani et al., 2012). This method produces good results providing the paper surface is not too rough – which has the effect of making the hills difficult to distinguish from the valleys.

10.7   Miscellaneous factors

There are many other possible ways in which a document can be dated depending on its nature.

- Pre-printed documents such as letterheads or invoices. These are often produced in batches and there may be variation between batches such as a printing defect of the kind described in Chapter 5, or slight differences in ink colour. Any features that can establish between-batch variations have the potential to assist with a dating problem, providing the relevant background information is available such as when batches were produced at the printers.

- Some items bear dates of production. Envelopes often bear such a date on an inner surface of the envelope. Envelopes also often have printed designs on them and these designs may be changed periodically, so again there is scope for determining when a particular envelope was first produced.

- Official documents, such as driving licences, undergo periodic revision. The dates of revision are often shown on the document.

- Changes to telephone numbers occur infrequently, such as revision to the dialling codes used in particular places. When such changes occur, this often leads to new pre-printed company documentation being needed.

- The introduction of any official changes may be relevant, such as the use of postcodes to address posted mail.

10.8   Summary

Backdating a document, particularly if it is many years later, is fraught with problems since it may be that the relevant batches of document are no longer available or the fact that telephone numbers have changed in the meantime is missed, or any of the other pitfalls described in this chapter have occurred. Such issues have been a significant component of the means by which a number of fraudulent documents have been exposed over the years.

In a slightly different context, fraudulent artwork shares many of the kinds of problems associated with documents, such as acquiring the appropriate materials relevant to a particular time when genuine art was produced by a given artist, and that is before the art is to be created in the correct and convincing manner expected of the artist concerned.

10.9   Case notes and reports in cases involving document dating

The method of dating a document will vary depending on which aspect(s) of the case were relevant. Thus it is not possible to generalise how case notes should be made or how the findings should be reported. However, dating is generally done either by an *absolute* process (such as showing when some paper was made by reference to manufacturing records, for example) or by a *relative* process (such as showing that a writer's signature deteriorated over time due to illness). In both situations, it is necessary to place the questioned document into a chronology that has been established by relevant information and thus a description of that chronology and the means for establishing it must form a part of the report. Then the placement of the disputed document into that chronology can be described so that the reader can understand how the document was dated.

Worked example

The examination types that are typically used are described in the relevant chapters and for this reason a worked example is not relevant to this chapter.

References

Aginsky, V. N. (1993). Some new ideas for dating ballpoint inks – a feasibility study. *Journal of Forensic Sciences*, 38(5), 1134–1150.

Allen, M. J., & Rimmer, P. A. (1988). The dating of a will. *Journal of the Forensic Science Society*, 28(3), 199–203. doi: 10.1016/S0015-7368(88)72830-3.

Cantu, A. A. (2012). A study of the evaporation of a solvent from a solution-application to writing ink aging. *Forensic Science International*, 219(1–3) doi:10.1016/j.forsciint .2011.12.008.

Ezcurra, M., Gongora, J. M. G., Maguregui, I., & Alonso, R. (2010). Analytical methods for dating modern writing instrument inks on paper. *Forensic Science International*, 197(1–3), 1–20. doi:10.1016/j.forsciint.2009.11.013.

Hardcastle, R. A. (1986). Progressive damage to plastic printwheel typing elements. *Forensic Science International*, 30(4), 267–274.

Li, B., Xie, P., Guo, Y., & Fei, Q. (2014). GC analysis of black gel pen ink stored under different conditions. *Journal of Forensic Sciences*, 59(2), 543–549. doi:10.1111/1556-4029 .12313.

Mathyer, J., & Pfister, R. (1984). The determination of sequence of crossing strokes by the kromekote paper lifting process and by the scanning electron-microscopic method. *Forensic Science International*, 24(2), 113–124. doi:10.1016/0379-0738(84)90091-4.

Montani, I., Mazzella, W., Guichard, M., & Marquis, R. (2012). Examination of heterogeneous crossing sequences between toner and rollerball pen strokes by digital microscopy and 3-D laser profilometry. *Journal of Forensic Sciences*, 57(4), 997–1002. doi:10.1111/j.1556-4029.2012.02103.x.

Ozbek, N., Braz, A., Lopez-Lopez, M., & Garcia-Ruiz, C. (2014). A study to visualize and determine the sequencing of intersecting ink lines. *Forensic Science International*, 234, 39–44. doi:10.1016/j.forsciint.2013.10.026.

Raza, A., & Saha, B. (2013). Application of raman spectroscopy in forensic investigation of questioned documents involving stamp inks. *Science & Justice*, 53(3), 332–338. doi:10.1016/j.scijus.2012.11.001.

Saini, K., Kaur, R., & Sood, N. C. (2009). Determining the sequence of intersecting gel pen and laser printed strokes - a comparative study. *Science & Justice*, 49(4), 286–291. doi:10.1016/j.scijus.2009.07.003.

Totty, R. N., Rimmer, P. A., & Steadman, R. K. (1987). Establishing the date of manufacture of a sheet of photocopy paper – a case example. *Journal of the Forensic Science Society*, 27(2), 81–88. doi: 10.1016/S0015-7368(87)72713-3.

Weyermann, C., Almog, J., Buegler, J., & Cantu, A. A. (2012). Minimum requirements for application of ink dating methods based on solvent analysis in casework (vol 210, pg 52, 2011). *Forensic Science International*, 214(1–3), 214–214. doi:10.1016/j.forsciint .2011.07.051.

Xu, Y., Wang, J., & Yao, L. (2006). Dating the writing age of black roller and gel inks by gas chromatography and UV-vis spectrophotometer. *Forensic Science International*, 162(1–3), 140–143. doi: 10.1016/j.forsciint.2006.06.011.

11
Duties of The Expert

Judicial systems vary from place to place. There are two models for hearings in court that predominate, namely the adversarial system where one side challenges another (typified by the UK) and the inquisitorial system where proceedings are focused on establishing 'the truth' (typified in much of the rest of Europe). This chapter will tend to focus on issues that relate to the adversarial system, but most of the principles apply to both systems of justice.

In addition, the system in the UK is split into two main subdivisions, namely the criminal and the civil courts. Hearings may take place outside the court's judicial system but the standards of proof almost always are modelled on the criminal (beyond reasonable doubt) or the civil (on the balance of probability) evidence requirements.

The giving of evidence in person is the final stage of the journey from the event to the judicial process of seeking to prove innocence, guilt, exoneration or blame of some kind. Of the many steps along the path, some are outside the control of the forensic expert, but once the evidence is available to examine, the responsibility lies with the expert to make sure that not only are the forensic processes carried out properly but also that the results obtained are made available in a clear and understandable way to the non-experts who need to fully understand them in the court proceedings or hearing that may follow.

For this reason, the importance of good written communication and good oral communication cannot be overstated despite coming as the final chapter of this book that focuses primarily on the forensic methods used in the speciality of document examination. Put quite simply, being expert at the forensic examinations involved and interpreting the results is all well and good, but if the end product (be it a report or giving verbal evidence in person) is incomprehensible or misleading then all that skill will come to nought.

Foundations of Forensic Document Analysis: Theory and Practice, First Edition. Michael Allen.
© 2016 John Wiley & Sons, Ltd. Published 2016 by John Wiley & Sons, Ltd.
Companion Website: www.wiley.com/go/allen/forensicanalysis

11.1   Note taking

The need to make thorough notes has been stressed throughout this book. The kinds of information needed for various examination types have been discussed when necessary as it is often the case that the details that need to be recorded are not obvious, since it is not practical to make a note of absolutely everything that occurs during an examination. Rather, it is more efficient if the notes contain the observations that are relevant to, and which form the basis of, any conclusions that are to be expressed in a final report.

At the time of making an examination it may not be obvious which observations, results, findings and overall thought processes are the most important for what will eventually go into the report. Hence, notes nearly always contain more information than appears in the final report, since the context of the case will dictate what is relevant and the reader of the report will not understand all of the many specialist, technical components of the notes.

It is therefore certainly true that the notes are primarily for the practitioner as an aide memoire of what was done and what was thought at the time of the examination such that, should it be necessary to give evidence in person at some later time, the essential elements of the forensic case are clear. However, there is perhaps a sense in which the notes are rather more than a personal record and are a public document, in that the evidence forthcoming from an examination is usually in the public domain, so it is wise to ensure that the notes are appropriate and have the potential to be scrutinised by others as being a good and fit for purpose record of the events of the examination – and that the practitioner did not do a superficial job, making inadequate case notes to back up the conclusions expressed.

One aspect of case file management that is important to note is ensuring the pagination of the many sheets of paper, with a note made of the total number of pages present. This enables the completeness and the presence of all material in the file to be demonstrated – missing pages or tampering with the file then become more obvious. Tampering with the file (for example removing or re-writing pages) could well call into question the integrity of the expert if discovered.

Often the case file can become very large, containing pages of notes, findings, perhaps printouts from various pieces of equipment and copies of one or more statements or reports. Given that the case file is the source of all of the relevant information about the case when it comes to court months or years after the examination(s) took place, it then becomes important that the contents of the file are organised in such a way as to ensure that retrieval of details can be done efficiently in the witness box in response to a question. There are many ways of making file navigation as clear as possible depending on the nature of the contents. Some suggestions include:

- If many items have been submitted then tabulate the exhibit references that they have against the pages (another advantage of pagination) on which case notes regarding each item were made. For example:

Item	Pages in notes
AB/2	2–4
GH/1	6 and 14

- If more than one report or statement has been written, place the report at the start followed by the pages of notes that are covered by that report together, and flag up each report in chronological order so that it can be found quickly.

- It is often best to put all of the administrative documentation (such as the submission form outlining what the investigator wanted and any documents relating to housekeeping of the case, such as time sheets) on one side of the file and the case notes on the other side. If more than one submission has been made in a case, it is best if they too are filed in chronological sequence.

Inefficient file navigation may not seem all that important to the forensic evidence (and indeed it has no bearing on it at all), but the perception of the court of an expert's competence might be adversely affected if after each question at a hearing there is a shuffling of papers lasting too long, such that the flow of oral evidence is disrupted. When onlookers wonder whether the expert can't keep their file in order, what does that say about the expert?

11.2 Reports

In those cases where, for one reason or another, the expert is not required to give evidence in person at a hearing, the report or statement is the final product of a forensic practitioner's task. If indeed their evidence is alluded to in a hearing in their absence, then it is crucial that the report's meaning is crystal clear since the expert is not there to correct any misapprehensions about what is being said in it.

It is not necessary for a forensic practitioner's report to be a literary master-piece. Indeed, it is important that it is straightforward and easy to understand by a non-expert. Some suggestions are:

- Simplicity is a crucial element of a forensic report, not to be confused with dumbing down (which seeks to remove any complexity from the subject being written about, rendering its content of less value).

- The use of jargon should be kept to a minimum but if it cannot be avoided then a glossary of terms might assist as long as it is not so extensive that it disrupts the reading of the report. An alternative is to put a very short explanation for any unfamiliar terms in brackets immediately after the term is used.

- The use of statistics in document examination reports is rarely needed. Any numerical evaluation of evidence is generally best 'translated' into a word-based equivalent. The main aim is to get the strength of evidence understood and, in particular, to identify any limitations to the evidence and the effect they have on the degree of certainty that can be expressed.

- Long and complex reports can be broken up into sections that have common themes. For example, it may help if all of the handwriting findings are reported in one section and the printing findings in another section and so on. Section headings and the use of summaries where relevant will all help to make the report more readily understood.

- The use of diagrams or photographs may assist when it is hard to explain a finding using words only.

- Often a reader will want to know the 'bottom line' of a report's findings before going on to read more of the details as to the whys and wherefores. This can be achieved by including an overall summary that contains a brief review of each of the findings about which more detail can be found in the body of the report.

The value of a well-written report to the reader is obvious, but the expert will also benefit because the likelihood of being called to give evidence in person may be reduced if the meaning of the report is clear to all concerned. In addition, if giving evidence in person, locating relevant findings will be quicker if the report is well structured. The written findings, conclusions and opinions are the basis for the oral evidence.

11.2.1 Expressing conclusions

Perhaps the most important aspect of a report is the conclusions. The ways in which they are expressed have the potential to have a significant impact on how a case will be judged. For this reason, much has been written over the years advocating different views on how this should be done to ensure that those who use the report in their deliberations understand clearly the strength of evidence that is available.

One part of this is the distinction between opinion evidence and factual evidence. The giving of opinion evidence is the territory of the expert witness. Giving factual evidence may also fall within the remit of the expert, but it may also be given by a professional witness whose expertise is in the relevant subject area. The demarcation between opinion and factual evidence is not always clear and legal distinctions between them may be debatable. Many conclusions are a hybrid of factual evidence and opinion evidence, but with some specialities the opinion element is greater than others, none more so than handwriting evidence which relies so heavily on the skill, experience and knowledge of the expert to interpret what are always unique examinations.

Notwithstanding philosophical subtleties, the expert is duty bound to say what he or she thinks the evidence that they have discovered means; simply revealing or describing the evidence without saying what it means falls short of expert evidence as it clearly leaves out any sort of interpretation. The interpretation of evidence is often dependent on the case story and this is why considering alternative explanations for it is so important. It is most certainly not the role of the expert to attempt to provide support for a particular interpretation of the evidence; rather, the unbiased expert will consider reasonable explanations in a given case and (giving reasons) will explain why one or other of the explanations better accounts for the findings than others.

11.3 Preparing for court

The time lapse between a forensic examination and attendance at a hearing in person may be months or even years. The case file then becomes the starting point for re-acquaintance with the case and the story behind it. Reading the case file is essential and it may well help if it can be established with the relevant authorities which parts of the evidence will be pertinent, since it is by no means unusual for only a part of an expert's evidence to be alluded to during the hearing. In such a situation, the expert can then concentrate on those elements of the case notes and reports that are relevant to the hearing, which is especially helpful if there was a lot of other material examined which is not relevant and can be ignored (or at least briefly skimmed over) in preparation for the hearing.

It may be possible to memorise much of the information in a smaller case, although it is always wise to check with the written notes first before answering questions during a hearing. In larger cases, it may only be possible to memorise a fairly small part of the information, so instead it is a good strategy to remember where various kinds of information are located in the file. If the case file has been constructed carefully (see previous section), then the retrieval of information required for an answer will be less difficult. Obviously, memory is an attribute that varies from person to person, so it is best to use one's own particular memory faculty to the best advantage.

Typically, experts will receive plenty of warning (weeks or months) before being required to give evidence in person, although it is not unknown for an expert's evidence to unexpectedly become relevant during a hearing and then the warning time may be days or hours! The place where the hearing is taking place is usually known well in advance, although again it can change at short notice since by their very nature hearings are unpredictable events and can take much less or much more time than anticipated.

Therefore, it is important to plan travel arrangements and to have a local map so that getting to a hearing is as swift and uneventful as possible. It is also important to have relevant contact details so that if travel is slow those at the hearing can be made aware of your delay. The time that a witness eventually gets to give evidence in person is often difficult to predict at the start of the day, so in most cases it is required that a witness be at the hearing at the start of a day's proceedings. Inevitably, this means that, even for expert witnesses, there is a good chance that there will be several hours waiting to give evidence (and it is not unusual to have to return the next day and even the next). It follows that it is worth having some means of passing the time.

Giving evidence is a generally stressful experience for a witness, even for an experienced expert witness. Some adrenalin is good to keep you on your toes as opposed to the opposite, complacency, which can make you feel over-confident. The impact of the evidence cannot be detached from the personality of the person giving it since we all react to people in different ways. How those at a hearing perceive a given expert witness is difficult to know, but some qualities that an expert might do well to show are:

- A lack of bias. Expert witnesses should be impartial and at no time should they appear to be slanting or selecting the evidence in favour of any party in a case.

- A willingness to reconsider. One symptom of bias is an unwillingness to either reconsider one's evidence (in the absence of any further information) or to consider other specific suggestions that might account for an expert's findings. A closed mind is a very dangerous position for an expert witness to take. Not only will those listening be concerned that the expert is either biased or over-confident, but even if the expert's evidence is in fact correct, it may not be believed for those very reasons.

- Humility. An expert witness is an important witness but that is not a reason to be self-important. This links to a willingness to reconsider, since no person is immune from error or misjudgement no matter how experienced and knowledgeable they are. That does not mean to say that experts are always wrong – they are not because they are extremely well informed and able to offer their experience and opinion to assist the court to the very best of their ability and in light of methods and knowledge at that time. Many people often find this simple and obvious truth unnerving since forensic seems to suggest perfect, incontrovertible evidence, especially if the word science is added in. These are important issues and an expert would do well to be prepared for the question: Do you ever make mistakes?

- Confidence in the sense of being sure of one's subject and having a firm grasp of the technical and interpretive aspects of the speciality without being dogmatic in its application.

Those listening to an expert's evidence will almost certainly have expectations of not only the manner in which the expert delivers this but also their behavioural demeanour and appearance. In this sense there is a degree of fulfilling the expectations of others by having a smart appearance and conducting oneself in and outside the hearing in a professional way.

Unfortunately, the one group of people that is often portrayed as being expected to be infallible is the experts. As noted elsewhere in this chapter, such an expectation is completely unreasonable, but experts should be doing everything within their personal capability and that of their speciality at that time (after all science, technology and methods do develop and should improve over time).

There is clearly a difference between an accidental error, an error caused by negligent practice and an error caused by corrupt practice. Errors of the first kind will happen but the likelihood is reduced when the expert is properly trained, keeps up to date with developments in their speciality (usually known as continuing professional development or CPD) and ideally has colleagues who are able to check their work to yet further reduce sources of error.

Errors of the second kind will tend to occur if the expert is not fully competent or has a disorganised and unprofessional approach to casework. While they are unacceptable they are capable of remediation with the help of further training and greater awareness of good practice.

Errors of the third kind, if revealed, should have only one consequence and that is that the expert is not able to practice.

11.4   Giving evidence

Speaking in public is something that many people find uncomfortable. In most hearings, the 'audience' is not especially large (typically 20 to 30 people perhaps) but the fact that the expert is giving evidence means that it is important evidence that requires the scrutiny that comes from clarification and challenge.

The giving of evidence requires that the expert is able to present information in a straightforward and clear way so that non-experts can understand what is being said and what conclusions are being drawn and that there is an understandable and reasonable link leading to the conclusions. To do this orally in front of others is not always an easy task. However, experts are obviously well versed with their subject matter. The more difficult part is using language that conveys the evidence without distorting or misrepresenting it. It is likely that experts will have undergone training in preparation for a career that requires giving oral evidence. From this the expert can build up a 'library' of responses to some of the more frequently encountered questions in their speciality. As the expert's experience increases, it is also possible to begin to anticipate which lines of questioning are more likely in a given case.

11.4.1   Giving your evidence

The pattern of giving evidence will vary from place to place, but often it involves two main stages. First, giving your evidence, which can include clarifying and adding explanations to it, and which also often starts with a general background scoping the speciality and its associated methods. Second, it is common for there to be some sort of challenge to the evidence to test it and justify it so that those listening to it can be reassured as to its quality.

In a sense, therefore, the first stage is usually more predictable and 'friendly' in that it is an opportunity for the expert to articulate his or her evidence for the benefit of the hearing so that it is clearly understood; the general principles are outlined and the observations in the particular case are related in such a way as to make a coherent and comprehensible story.

11.4.2   Answering questions

Challenging the evidence is necessary to ensure that the expert's evidence is credible. The challenge can be to the various components of the evidence itself:

- The speciality itself – are the methods and knowledge underpinning it reliable?

- The observations, measurements, interpretations and conclusions in the particular case.

- The expert's competence.

The need for forensic specialities to be founded on sound principles was discussed in Chapter 1. Chapters 2–10 contain much of the information that both underpins the speciality of forensic document examination and also describes the kinds of observations and their interpretation for various examination types. Various means have been put forward to reassure users of forensic evidence over the competence of experts and these are also described in Chapter 1.

The expert can expect to be challenged on any or all of these aspects. If the speciality has a long, tried and tested history, then it is unlikely that this will be significantly challenged. If the expert has done his or her job properly and explained things well, then this will make a challenge to the case findings more difficult. Direct 'attacks' on expert witnesses are unusual but having some form of external backup to demonstrate competence helps to give confidence to the listener.

Questions that challenge the forensic evidence are often the most difficult to answer. It is always good practice to think carefully before any answer is given since retracting an answer is not easy. This is particularly true if the answer required is not just a simple yes or no, but requires an explanation that is coherent and understandable.

If new material is produced for an expert during a hearing then it is wise to require time to consider it carefully – examinations made in the witness box (such as a new document bearing handwriting and the question 'Was this written by the same person as the other documents you have seen?' or some such situation) are generally unwise unless given with the caveat that they are first impressions.

It is often the case that at least some parts of your evidence will be written down manually by people in the hearing as you speak (and all of it will be recorded in some way). This means that if the witness speaks too quickly, those noting your words may ask for an answer to be repeated or a general slowing down in speaking speed. This may sound straightforward enough, but people have a natural tempo for their speech and changing it can be difficult.

The questioner is not usually an expert in questioned documents and so may either inadvertently or deliberately ask questions the meaning of which is not clear to you (and therefore almost certainly not clear to the others at the hearing). It is wise to have the question re-phrased to make sure that you have understood it correctly and at the same time make clear to those listening to your answer the connection between question and answer.

Taking time over answering, especially if the question is either unexpected, or complex or perhaps seems particularly important to your evidence, is a good policy. It is expected that an expert will answer questions with due careful thought when needed. And there is most certainly no requirement that an expert's answer should be constrained by such comments as 'Just answer Yes or No' if such an answer is inappropriate.

11.5   Ethics and duties of experts

The single most important guiding rule for expert witnesses is to ensure that nothing they do impedes fairness and justice. In other words, their duty is to the court (and therefore ultimately to society as a whole). This may be a heavy burden to bear given that some of the other players in the judicial system are not averse to suppressing, misrepresenting or slanting evidence. But expert witnesses should seek to take the highest possible moral high ground in the way they conduct themselves in all aspects of their business, from the time that they take on a case to the time they are giving oral evidence.

11.5.1   Dealing with clients

Dealings with a client fall into two broad categories. There is the forensic side that involves the technical matters about which the expert has been consulted. But there is also the business side in which factors such as cost and timeliness are relevant.

The expert must examine all of the material that they are presented with and must not select evidence that supports their client's (or anyone else's) case – this would be clearly wrong. It may be true that the adversarial system in particular leans towards the mentality of 'prove it', but the expert must be above that and must consider all evidence presented to them. Indeed, it is certainly possible that those supplying the evidence may already have selected items for examination that they believe help their cause (and possibly *not* supplied material that they believe will be detrimental to their case) and that is something that may well not be apparent or known to the expert.

It is often the case that clients will not like the expert's report if it does not say what they wanted or expected it to say. Experts may be asked to re-consider their conclusions, and that can be done, but change can only be justified on the available evidence not because of the client's say so. An expert may be asked to leave out particularly damaging parts of their report and, again, this interference must not be tolerated.

One occurrence that presents especially awkward problems is where an instructing client asks for a particular aspect of a questioned document case to be examined and does not ask for (and potentially will not pay for) other aspects of the document to be examined – either because they are not aware that those other aspects can be examined or because they know what the outcome will be and do not want that revealed. If the expert carries out the requested examination but also notices that an unrequested aspect could be relevant to the case as a whole (although perhaps damaging to the client's case), what should be done? Opinions on this may differ, but if fairness and justice are the primary duty of the expert, then this unrequested aspect must at least be brought out into the open by some appropriate means so that the conscience of the expert is clear even if others choose not to pursue it. It does not help matters when client confidentiality is invoked as a barrier to what an expert can or should do. As noted above, expert witnesses are responsible ultimately to the courts, and they should take the highest possible moral standpoint and behave accordingly and should not be criticised or threatened with legal consequences for doing so.

Experts do have a business side to their jobs and it is right that this too is carried out in a professional way. It is to be hoped that experts that do not deliver their services in a timely way or unreasonably over-charge, for example, will not stay in business.

It may be that experts face some difficult issues over the way in which they charge their clients. It is not unknown for an expert to provide their services for free if the client is clearly unable to (fully) pay and if there is a good reason to believe that there is something of potential importance that needs expert examination. At the opposite end of the spectrum are clients for whom paying is not an issue and who are prepared to pay a premium, especially for a faster service for example. Such business practices are normal, but one that is not to be encouraged is the so-called 'no win, no fee', which translates into the expert not charging if the client does not win the case. In such circumstances, the expert would have a vested financial interest in the outcome of the case which could (and almost certainly would be seen by others to) compromise the unbiased nature of the expert's evidence.

11.5.2 Cognitive bias

It must be remembered that for a variety of reasons experts may be given background information by one or other party to a case and may even be told that, for example, a specimen of handwriting was written by a particular person when in fact it was not. Such background information may be necessary to a case in that it enables the expert to consider the various alternative possibilities, but it may also influence their examination and conclusion along the lines of 'X has admitted writing the document so it is safe for me to reach that conclusion' when crucially that conclusion may not be justified on the basis of the evidence available. This tendency (known as cognitive bias) to make the evidence consistent with the 'known (or believed) facts' is extremely dangerous, turns the whole forensic process upside down and is quite simply wrong.

Cognitive bias may be difficult to deal with when the investigator has a very strong expectation of an outcome from a forensic examination, and this may be exacerbated if the case has a particularly high media profile often resulting from a major incident. The pressure on the expert to deliver the anticipated or even 'needed' result must at all costs be resisted. Rather, the evidence must be evaluated in the normal way using all of the methods and processes required and interpreted according to the normal criteria that would apply to any other case.

This also highlights a drawback to an organisational relationship between the investigator and the expert. If the expert works for the same organisation as the investigator, then there is a danger that either the expert will feel under pressure to occasionally provide the result expected by a particularly keen (but unwise) investigator, or that others will perceive the investigator–expert relationship as too close and will call into question the expert's impartiality no matter how independent-minded the expert really is. This is not calling into question the expert's integrity, but makes the point that others may be sceptical of it.

Cognitive bias can occur when one expert checks another expert's work as there may be a tendency for the checker to only look at the points that led the first expert to their conclusion. This is not a wise approach to quality assurance checking. Having made their own independent examination and formed a conclusion, it is essential that the checker should challenge the evidence of the first expert, looking for errors, inconsistencies, and essentially putting into practice one of the cornerstones of scientific method, namely trying to falsify (or trying to show as incorrect) the reported findings and conclusions. If the checker cannot find reasons to undermine the report's conclusions then it is reasonable to accept them as a fair representation of the evidence.

Experts should neither believe nor disbelieve what they are told by others in a case as people have all sorts of reasons for admitting and denying things, either by deliberately lying or in the mistaken belief that what they are saying is true. Experts have to work on the *presumption* that some of what they are told is true (such as Person X attended and provided the sample of hand-writing submitted) but they must be aware that some of what they are told may not be true and should, if possible, test any such information if the evidence is available. For example, if a person admits all of the handwriting in a diary, but the expert finds clear evidence that there is the handwriting of more than one person present, that has to be made clear in any report even though it may not be possible for the expert to establish which, *if any*, of the multiple handwritings in the diary were written by the person making the admission.

11.6 Summary

There are, therefore, many non-technical aspects to the work of the forensic document examiner that are not optional but must be dealt with properly and professionally. These aspects can indeed reflect on the integrity and business capability of an expert and have the potential to cause as much damage to an expert's reputation as competence in the speciality itself. In general, openness, transparency and honesty combined with a clear awareness of where duties lie will be sufficient to avoid the majority of awkward professional situations that can arise.

Index

Foundations of Forensic Document Analysis: Theory and Practice, First Edition. Michael Allen.
© 2016 John Wiley & Sons, Ltd. Published 2016 by John Wiley & Sons, Ltd.
Companion Website: www.wiley.com/go/allen/forensicanalysis